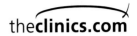

SURGICAL CLINICS
OF NORTH AMERICA

Gastric Surgery

GUEST EDITOR
Ronald F. Martin, MD

CONSULTING EDITOR
Ronald F. Martin, MD

October 2005 • Volume 85 • Number 5

SAUNDERS

An Imprint of Elsevier, Inc.
PHILADELPHIA   LONDON   TORONTO   MONTREAL   SYDNEY   TOKYO

W.B. SAUNDERS COMPANY
A Division of Elsevier Inc.

1600 John F. Kennedy Blvd., Suite 1800, Philadelphia, PA 19103-2899

http://www.theclinics.com

SURGICAL CLINICS OF NORTH AMERICA
October 2005
Editor: Catherine Bewick

Volume 85, Number 5
ISSN 0039–6109
ISBN 1-4160-2794-7

Reprints. For copies of 100 or more of articles in this publication, please contact the commercial Reprints Department Elsevier Inc., 360 Park Avenue South, New York, New York 10010-1710. Tel. (212) 633-3813, Fax: (212) 462-1935, email: reprints@elsevier.com

The ideas and opinions expressed in *The Surgical Clinics of North America* do not necessarily reflect those of the Publisher. The Publisher does not assume any responsibility for any injury and/or damage to persons or property arising out of or related to any use of the material contained in this periodical. The reader is advised to check the appropriate medical literature and the product information currently provided by the manufacturer of each drug to be administered to verify the dosage, the method and duration of administration, or contraindications. It is the responsibility of the treating physician or other health care professional, relying on independent experience and knowledge of the patient, to determine drug dosages and the best treatment for the patient. Mention of any product in this issue should not be construed as endorsement by the contributors, editors, or the Publisher of the product or manufacturers' claims.

Surgical Clinics of North America (ISSN 0039–6109) is published bimonthly by Elsevier; Corporate and editorial Offices: 1600 John F. Kennedy Blvd., Suite 1800, Philadelphia, PA 19103-2899. Accounting and circulation offices: 6277 Sea Harbor Drive, Orlando, FL 32887-4800. Periodicals postage paid at Orlando, FL 32862, and additional mailing offices. Subscription prices are $190.00 per year for US individuals, $299.00 per year for US institutions, $95.00 per year for US students and residents, $234.00 per year for Canadian individuals, $365.00 per year for Canadian institutions, $250.00 for international individuals, $365.00 for international institutions and $125.00 per year for Canadian and foreign students/residents. To receive student/resident rate, orders must be accompanied by name of affiliated institution, date of term, and the *signature* of program/residency coordinator on institution letterhead. Orders will be billed at individual rate until proof of status is received. Foreign air speed delivery is included in all *Clinics* subscription prices. All prices are subject to change without notice. POSTMASTER: Send address changes to *The Surgical Clinics of North America*, W.B. Saunders Company, Periodicals Fulfillment, Orlando, FL 32887-4800. **Customer Service: 1-800-654-2452 (US). From outside of the US, call 1-407-345-1000.**

The Surgical Clinics of North America is also published in Spanish by McGraw-Hill Interamericana Editores S.A., P.O. Box 5-237 06500 Mexico D.F. Mexico; and in Portuguese by Interlivros Edicoes Ltda., Rua Comandante Coelho 1085, CEP 21250, Rio de Janeiro, Brazil; and in Greek by Paschalidis Medical Publications, Athens Greece.

The Surgical Clinics of North America is covered in *Index Medicus*, *EMBASE/Excerpta Medica*, *Current Contents/Clinical Medicine*, *Current Contents/Life Sciences*, *Science Citation Index*, and *ISI/BIOMED*.

Printed in the United States of America.

CONSULTING EDITOR

RONALD F. MARTIN, MD, Department of Surgery, Marshfield Clinic and Saint Joseph's Hospital, Marshfield, Wisconsin; Clinical Associate Professor of Surgery, University of Vermont, Burlington, Vermont

GUEST EDITOR

RONALD F. MARTIN, MD, Department of Surgery, Marshfield Clinic and Saint Joseph's Hospital, Marshfield, Wisconsin; Clinical Associate Professor of Surgery, University of Vermont, Burlington, Vermont

CONTRIBUTORS

RICHARD H. BELL, Jr, MD, FACS, Loyal and Edith Davis Professor and Chair, Department of Surgery, Northwestern University Feinberg School of Medicine, Chicago, Illinois

JO BUYSKE, MD, Chief, Department of Surgery; Assistant Professor of Surgery, Penn Presbyterian Medical Center, Philadelphia, Pennsylvania

DERICK J. CHRISTIAN, MD, Instructor in Laparoscopic Surgery, Department of Surgery, Penn Presbyterian Medical Center, Philadelphia, Pennsylvania

ANDREW C. DUKOWICZ, MD, Fellow, Section of Gastroenterology and Hepatology; Instructor of Medicine, Dartmouth Medical School, Dartmouth Hitchcock Medical Center, Lebanon, New Hampshire

SHEILA ESWARAN, MD, Department of Medicine, Maine Medical Center, Portland, Maine

RICARDO J. GONZALEZ, MD, Fellow, Department of Surgical Oncology, The University of Texas MD Anderson Cancer Center, Houston, Texas

B. TODD HENIFORD, MD, FACS, Chief, Division of Gastrointestinal and Minimally Invasive Surgery, Carolinas Medical Center, Charlotte, North Carolina

BRIAN E. LACY, PhD, MD, Associate Professor of Medicine; Director, Gastrointestinal Motility Laboratory, Section of Gastroenterology and Hepatology, Dartmouth-Hitchcock Medical Center, Lebanon, New Hampshire

PAUL F. MANSFIELD, MD, FACS, Professor of Surgery, Department of Surgical Oncology, The University of Texas MD Anderson Cancer Center, Houston, Texas

RONALD F. MARTIN, MD, Department of Surgery, Marshfield Clinic and Saint Joseph's Hospital, Marshfield, Wisconsin; Clinical Associate Professor of Surgery, University of Vermont, Burlington, Vermont

J. LAWRENCE MUNSON, MD, Senior Staff Surgeon, Lahey Clinic Medical Center, Burlington, Massachusetts

RUTH O'MAHONY, MD, Lahey Clinic Medical Center, Burlington, Massachusetts

MICHAEL J. ROSEN, MD, Assistant Professor of Surgery, Case Western Reserve, Cleveland, Ohio

RICHARD I. ROTHSTEIN, MD, Chief, Section of Gastroenterology and Hepatology; Professor of Medicine, Dartmouth Medical School, Dartmouth Hitchcock Medical Center, Lebanon, New Hampshire

MICHAEL A. ROY, MD, Portland Gastroenterology Associates, Portland, Maine; Assistant Clinical Professor of Medicine, University of Vermont College of Medicine, Burlington, Vermont

DAVID I. SOYBEL, MD, Staff Surgeon, Department of Surgery, Brigham and Women's Hospital; Associate Professor of Surgery, Harvard Medical School, Boston, Massachusetts

JEFFREY D. WAYNE, MD, FACS, Assistant Professor of Surgery, Division of Surgical Oncology, Northwestern University Feinberg School of Medicine, Chicago, Illinois

KIRSTEN WEISER, MD, Fellow in Gastroenterology, Section of Gastroenterology and Hepatology, Dartmouth-Hitchcock Medical Center, Lebanon, New Hampshire

CONTENTS

gastroparesis are nonspecific. This article reviews normal and abnormal gastric motility, discusses the etiology and pathogenesis of gastroparesis, and provides an overview on new treatment options for gastroparesis, including gastric stimulation.

Endoluminal Gastric Surgery: the Modern Era of Minimally Invasive Surgery

Michael J. Rosen and B. Todd Heniford

Laparoendoluminal techniques are the next frontier in modern surgery. They provide a minimally invasive approach to gastric diseases that enables organ preservation while maintaining open surgical principles. Laparoscopic direct access to the stomach provides a magnified, high-resolution image for precise excision using widely available laparoscopic instrumentation. Further improvements in flexible endoscopic equipment, combined with the infusion of robotic instrumentation, will aid in overcoming the technical demands of this procedure and fuel the growth of endoluminal gastric surgery. Based on the currently available data, in appropriately selected patients, endoluminal gastric surgery affords the patients a definitive surgical procedure with all the advantages of a minimally invasive approach.

Limited Gastric Resection

Jeffrey D. Wayne and Richard H. Bell, Jr

Despite recent advancements in the staging and treatment of gastric cancer, overall survival remains poor. Extended or radical resections, to include the entire stomach, regional lymph nodes, or contiguous organs, have thus been proposed to alter the course of this fatal disease; however, no prospective randomized trial has validated this approach in a Western center. Furthermore, there are other malignant tumors that occur in the stomach and that may be successfully treated with a limited, nonanatomic, or subtotal gastrectomy, or in the case of gastric lymphoma, without surgery at all. Palliative approaches to patients who have advanced gastric cancer, which should be conservative by nature, are also outlined.

Radical Gastrectomy for Cancer of the Stomach

J. Lawrence Munson and Ruth O'Mahony

Carcinoma of the stomach remains one of the most common causes of cancer deaths in the world. The only treatment to offer hope for cure or long-term palliation is surgery. Optimal surgical resection requires an adequate margin of normal tissue around the tumor, dissection of perigastric lymph nodes, and en-bloc removal of organs involved by direct extension. Extended lymphadenectomy has not been shown to offer survival advantage in the West.

FORTHCOMING ISSUES

RECENT ISSUES

The Clinics are now available online!

www.theclinics.com

ELSEVIER
SAUNDERS

SURGICAL
CLINICS OF
NORTH AMERICA

Surg Clin N Am 85 (2005) xi–xii

Preface

Gastric Surgery

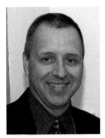

Ronald F. Martin, MD
Guest Editor

This issue of the *Surgical Clinics of North America* addresses the topic of gastric surgery. This topic relates to surgery in its truest sense. Surgery is a way of life, a state of mind and a discipline—occasionally, a passion. Although sometimes the word "surgery" is improperly used synonymously with "operation," the study of gastric surgery is an excellent reminder that our discipline requires a far broader understanding than that of mere technical matters. The contributors to this issue represent a wide variety of clinical interests and backgrounds. We have made an attempt to discuss the anatomic and physiologic principles that guide us in our management, as well as the operative issues in managing both malignant and benign conditions. The extent of operative management for neoplastic conditions from as limited as possible to radical resections is discussed, as is the operative management of benign conditions. In keeping with our belief that surgeons need to understand the disease processes of the stomach fully, we have included discussions of the medical management of neoplastic and benign conditions as well as motility disorders. And although some surgeons may consider it heresy, there is a discussion of endoscopic antireflux procedures.

I hope that the readers of this issue will find it a useful resource on its own merits, but also a starting point for further intellectual inquiry. Even a compilation of topics such as this can only begin to plumb the depths of knowledge and rich history of investigation and achievement upon which it is based.

I would like to thank all of the contributors greatly for their contributions to this issue. I would also like to thank Ms. Catherine Bewick, our publisher at Elsevier, for her tremendous commitment to this issue and the entire series. Without her support, this series would not be possible.

Ronald F. Martin, MD
Department of Surgery
Marshfield Clinic
1000 North Oak Avenue
Marshfield, WI 54449, USA

E-mail address: martin.ronald@marshfieldclinic.org

ELSEVIER
SAUNDERS

SURGICAL
CLINICS OF
NORTH AMERICA

Surg Clin N Am 85 (2005) 875–894

Anatomy and Physiology of the Stomach

David I. Soybel, MD

*Department of Surgery, Brigham and Women's Hospital, Harvard Medical School,
75 Francis Street Boston, MA 02115, USA*

Among the viscera, the stomach is among the earliest to have been described by priests, physicians, and anatomists and to have been studied functionally by alchemists, chemists, and physiologists [1–3]. The ancient Egyptians recognized the gross anatomy and the infirmity of the stomach; at the time of burial, it was preserved separately in one of the four so-called "canopic" jars (protected by the jackal god-son of Horus, Tuamutef). Hippocrates called digestion "pepsis," likening it to cooking, and proposing that the heat of the stomach was responsible for the breakdown of food [1].

A scientifically motivated understanding of gastric structure and function can be traced to 1547, when Andreas Vesalius, in his *De Humani Corporis Fabrica*, provided anatomically correct descriptions of the human stomach and intestines. In 1648, observations of animal digestion led J.B. van Helmont to postulate that different kinds of acids might play a role in digestion, calling them ferments [2]. In the 1780s, Lazzaro Spallanzani published his *Dissertationi de Fisica Animale e Vegetale*. This and his subsequent observations were works of extraordinary breadth and dedication to providing empirical distinction among fermentation (a chemical process of dissolution), digestion (the chemical process of dissolution produced by vital organs), and trituration (the mechanical process of foodstuff disintegration). Spallanzani had experimental subjects, including himself, swallow enclosed receptacles (linen bags or perforated metal tubes). He observed that, over time, the contents disappeared from the receptacle and postulated the involvement of acid [3,4]. In 1823, Prout, Tiedemann, and Gmelin each independently identified the acid in the stomach as hydrochloric acid [4]. International excitement and acclaim followed the publication in 1833, by the American army surgeon William Beaumont, of his *Observations on the Gastric Juice and the Physiology of Digestion*. Taking advantage of the opportunity to study human digestion through the portal of a gastro-cutaneous fistula in the

E-mail address: dsoybel@partners.org

young fur trapper, Alexis St. Martin, Beaumont persuasively confirmed the hypothesis that proper digestion requires the secretion of hydrochloric acid, observed evidence for an additional factor that permits putrefaction (pepsin?), and recognized changes in mucosal color and gastric motility in response to emotional disturbances or ingestion of strong spirits [5]. Beaumont is also generally credited with recognizing that secretion of digestive agents implies that the stomach has mechanisms for protecting itself from the damaging effects of its secretions [5], a physiologic principle not experimentally defined until the early 1960s in the work of Charles Code [6] and Horace Davenport [7].

Anatomy of the stomach

Landmarks

Topographically, the stomach has five regions (Fig. 1): (1) the cardia and gastroesophageal (GE) junction, (2) the fundus, (3) the corpus, (4) the antrum, and (5) the pylorus. The fundus and corpus harbor acid-secreting glands, whereas the antrum harbors alkaline-secreting surface epithelium and endocrine, gastrin-secreting G-cells. Viewed through a laparotomy incision or a laparoscope (Fig. 2), the GE junction is recognized at the sharp angle between the rounded dome of the fundus and the straight esophageal tube. The pylorus has no easily visualized landmarks, but is easily palpated as a ring of muscle separating the stomach and duodenum. Viewing the stomach externally, the junction between the acid-secreting corpus and the non-acid secreting antrum is identified on the lesser curvature by the incisura angularis.

Viewed endoscopically, the GE junction is easily distinguished by the transition between the flat, pale, stratified epithelium of the esophagus and

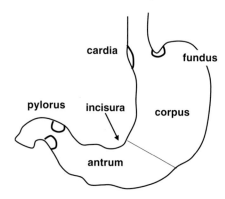

Fig. 1. Topography of the stomach.

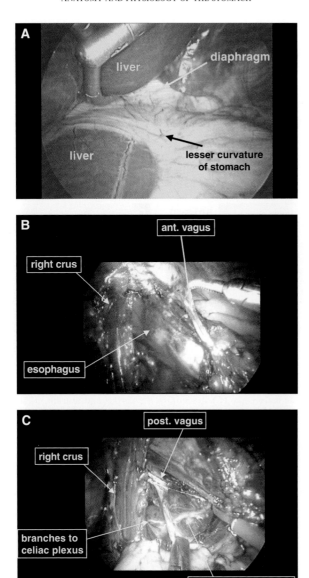

Fig. 2. Laparoscopic view of the stomach. (*A*) Anterior view. (*B*) GE junction, left crura, and anterior vagus. (*C*) Posterior vagus.

the lush, pink, glandular epithelium of the upper stomach (Fig. 3A, B). The junction between the acid-secreting corpus and the non-acid secreting antrum is also relatively easily distinguished by the rugal pattern: those of the antrum are linear and aligned with the long axis of the organ, whereas those of the corpus are convoluted and oriented obliquely (Fig. 3C). The

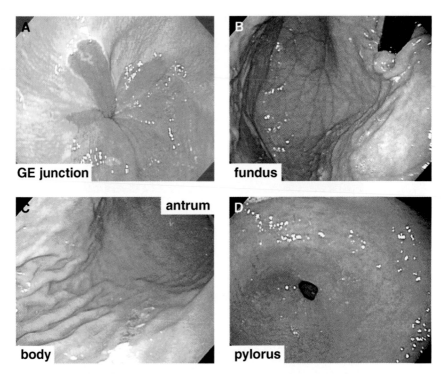

Fig. 3. Endoscopic view of the stomach. (*A*) GE junction. (*B*) Fundus viewed by means of retroflexion of the endoscope. (*C*) Junction of the corpus and antrum, noting the transition from obliquely oriented rugae to a relatively flat mucosa. (*D*) Pylorus.

pylorus is also easily visualized, outlined by the underlying ring of muscularis (Fig. 3D).

In the elderly, the non-acid secreting mucosa of the antrum may migrate cephalad, replacing acid-secreting mucosa in association with up to a 30% decrease in functional acid-secreting capacity [8–10]. Loss of oxyntic mucosa is likely due to the presence of chronic gastritis [8,10], increasing the area of gastrin-secreting mucosa and also altering the region of decreased resistance where gastric ulcers tend to arise (within 2 to 3 cm of the corpus/antrum junction) [11]. These are important considerations in choosing the boundaries of distal gastric resection for peptic ulcer disease.

Anatomic relationships

At the GE junction, the anatomic relationships include the diaphragm and crura (Figs. 4 and 5). Laterally, the cardiac notch signals a cardiac fat pad that must be released to expose the left crura. At the level of the fundus and proximal corpus, which are oriented vertically, the spleen is lateral and the lateral segment of the left lobe is medial and anterior (see Figs. 4 and 5).

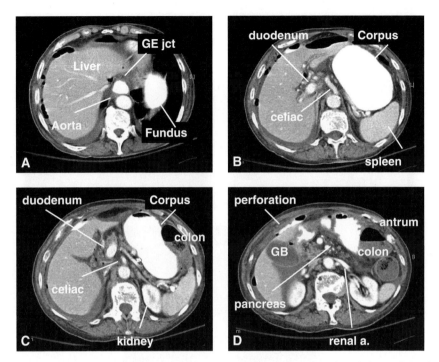

Fig. 4. CT images of the stomach—transverse sections. (A) Relationships of the cardia and fundus. (B) Relationships in the proximal corpus. (C) Relationships in the distal corpus, at the level of the celiac axis and the splenic artery. (D) Relationships of the antrum and pyloris. In this panel, the patient has a duodenal perforation in the duodenal bulb.

Posteriorly and medially lies the abdominal aorta, after being transmitted from the thorax through the diaphragm. Importantly, if the left lobe must be mobilized to expose the GE junction or proxima lesser curvature, the triangular ligament of the left hepatic lobe is incised, but not so far to the left as to injure the branch of the left inferior phrenic vein that passes in front of the esophageal hiatus toward the inferior vena cava, anteriorly and to the right.

The incisura signals the junction of the distal corpus and antrum (see Fig. 3), which are oriented horizontally. At this level, the aorta passes directly posterior to the body of the pancreas, which is in turn directly posterior to the gastric antrum. The transverse colon hangs interiorly, and the splenic flexure lies laterally to the left. The fundus of the gallbladder hangs superior to the pylorus and duodenal bulb, and the common bile duct passes posterior to the duodenal bulb on its way into the head of the pancreas, ultimately to empty on the medial wall of the duodenum.

The greater omentum is suspended from the greater curvature of the stomach, and has largely avascular attachments to the hepatic flexure, transverse segment, and splenic flexure of the colon. The lesser omentum

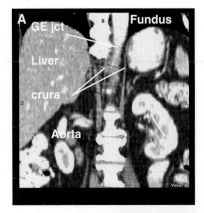
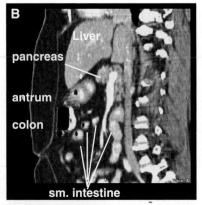

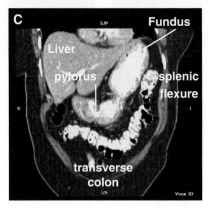

Fig. 5. Multiplanar views of the relationships of the stomach. (*A*) Coronal view of the GE junction and crura, spleen to the left and splenic flexure to the right and inferior. (*B*) Sagittal view of antrum. (*C*) Coronal view of stomach and transverse colon. (Courtesy of Peter Clark, MD, Department of Radiology, Brigham and Women's Hospital, Boston, MA.)

hangs between the lesser curvature of the stomach and a plane roughly connecting the falciform ligament. A portion of the lesser omentum, the pars flaccida, lies loosely near the lesser curvature and is a guidepost in morbid-obesity operations.

Arterial blood supply

The stomach is richly vascularized, with contributions from five major sources (Fig. 6): (1) the left gastric artery, a branch of the celiac axis, which supplies the cephalad portion of the lesser curvature; (2) the right gastric artery, a branch of the common hepatic artery, which supplies the caudal portion of the lesser curvature; (3) the right gastroepiploic artery, a branch of the gastroduodenal artery, which supplies the antrum and lower corpus; (4) the left gastroepiploic artery, a branch of the splenic artery, which

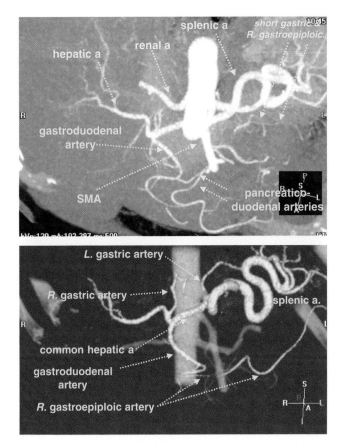

Fig. 6. Magnetic resonance arteriography (MRA) images of gastric vascular anatomy. (*Upper*) Maximum intensity projection (MIP) showing all branches of the celiac axis, with organs subtracted. (*Lower*) Three-dimensional projections to enhance vessels around the stomach, with attenuation of branches of hepatic artery and superior mesenteric artery. (Courtesy of Matthew Barish, MD, Department of Radiology, Brigham and Women's Hospital.)

supplies the upper corpus; and (5) a series of short gastric arteries passing to the fundus and cephalad portion of the corpus from the splenic hilum, and thus ultimately from the splenic artery. An inconstant branch to the pylorus has been also described, often as a branch of the gastroduodenal artery. On the lesser curvature, the left gastric artery does not always trace directly back from the lesser curvature to the celiac axis; in some cases it dips behind the body the pancreas before ascending posteriorly. On the greater curvature, there is a small bare area between the entrances of the right and left gastroepiploic into the gastric wall. This bare area serves as a useful landmark in identifying the proximal extent of the gastric antrum, corresponding to the incisura on the lesser curvature.

Innervation

The vagus nerves descend laterally along the esophagus; at the diaphragm they form the anterior and posterior vagal trunks (Fig. 7). At the level of the diaphragm, the anterior vagus is composed variably of one or two, and occasionally three, trunks adherent to the muscularis of the esophagus (Fig. 8) [12]. At the level of the GE junction, small branches pass through the anterior leaflet of the lesser omentum toward the liver and gallbladder; at this point, the vagal trunk becomes the anterior nerve of Latarjet. At this level, the posterior vagus is usually, but not always, a single trunk, passing the left side of the esophagus, bowing away from the lesser curvature. At the GE junction, small branches diverge to the right and posteriorly, and a sizeable branch is often observed angling sharply to the left to curl around the cardia (see Fig. 2C). In ulcer surgery, failure to recognize this latter branch, the so-called "criminal" nerve of Grassi, is thought to be responsible for some cases of incomplete vagotomy and subsequent recurrence of symptoms.

Lymphatic drainage

Lymphatic drainage pathways run in close proximity to the arterial supply (Fig. 9) [13]. A superior or left gastric group of nodes (between 10 and 20) lie along the cephalad lesser curvature and the left gastric artery. A suprapyloric group of nodes (3 to 6) lies along the lesser curvature and right gastric artery. The pancreaticosplenic group of nodes (3 to 5) drain the greater curvature along the fundus and upper corpus. Between 6 and 12 nodes lie along the right gastroepiploic artery. An additional subpyloric

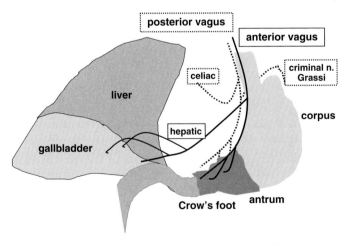

Fig. 7. Schematic illustration of the vagus and its branches as they descend along the greater curvature of the stomach.

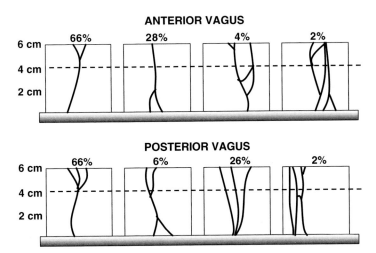

Fig. 8. Variations in anatomy of the anterior and posterior branches of the vagus nerves in the region of the GE junction and diaphragm. Incidence (%) of each anatomic group is indicated. (*Adapted from* Jackson RG. Anatomic Record 1949;103:1, 6; with permission.)

group of nodes (6 to 8) are identified at the pylorus and junction of the right gastroepiploic artery and gastroduodenal artery. Interconnections are numerous. For the purposes of staging of gastric carcinoma, 16 nodal stations have been distinguished, according to the Japanese Research Society for the study of Gastric Cancer (JRSGC). These stations are outlined in Table 1 [13], along with their designations as local (R1), regional (R2) or distal-regional (R3) spread.

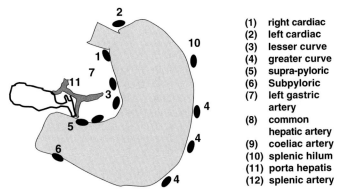

(1) right cardiac
(2) left cardiac
(3) lesser curve
(4) greater curve
(5) supra-pyloric
(6) Subpyloric
(7) left gastric artery
(8) common hepatic artery
(9) coeliac artery
(10) splenic hilum
(11) porta hepatis
(12) splenic artery

Fig. 9. Regional lymphatic drainage sites of the stomach, classified according to the Japanese Research Society for the Study of Gastric Cancer (JRSGC). (*From* Jpn J Surg 1981;11:127–39; with permission.)

Table 1
Stations of nodal spread in gastric cancer, classified according to the system of the Japanese
Research Society of study of Gastric Cancer

Station	Location	Antrum	Corpus/fundus
1	Right cardia	R2	R1
2	Left cardia	R2	R1
3	Lesser curve	R1	R2
4	Greater curve	R1	R2
5	Suprapyloric Right gastric a.	R1	R2
6	Infrapyloric	R1	R2
7	Left gastric a.	R1	R1
8	Common hepatic a.	R2	R2
9	Celiac axis	R3	R3
10	Splenic hilum	R3	R1
11	Splenic a.	R3	R1
12	Hepatoduodenal Ligament	R2	R1
13	Pancreas head	R2	R2
14	Root of SMA	R3	R3
15	Middle Colic a.	R3	R3
16	Para-aortic	R3	R3

From Jpn J Surg 1981;11:127–45; with permission.

Functional anatomy and physiology

The gastric mucosa

Functionally, the gastric mucosa is divided into acid-secreting and non-acid secreting regions. Acid- and pepsinogen-secreting mucosa is found in the corpus and fundus. The acid secreting unit of the mucosa is the gastric gland, schematically illustrated in Fig. 10. At the base of the gastric gland lie the pepsinogen-secreting chief cells. The middle of the gastric gland is populated largely with the HCl-secreting parietal cells. Toward the lumen, at the neck, parietal cells are still present, but give way to mucus neck cells and then, near the opening, the mucosa is largely populated with surface epithelial cells. Intercalated between parietal cells and smaller immature cells are enterochromaffin-like (ECL) cells expressing histidine decarboxylase, the enzyme that is essential in production of the paracrine agonist, histamine. The key features of the cell biology of acid secretion [14,15] are illustrated in Fig. 11, including its basis in ion transport (Fig. 11A), and in intracellular signaling stimulated by locally active neurohumoral agonists (Fig. 11B).

Neuroendocrine regulation of acid secretion

Three neurohumoral pathways figure prominently in the stimulation of acid secretion by the gastric mucosa [16]. These include: (1) acetylcholine, which is released by the vagus nerve; (2) histamine, released locally by ECL cells; and (3) gastrin, released by the gastric antrum and carried through the circulation to act on ECL cells and the parietal cells. As emphasized in

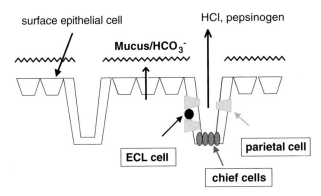

Fig. 10. Schematic illustration of the gastric mucosa, spatially and functionally divided into two regions: the acid-secreting gastric gland, and the mucus-alkali secreting surface epithelium. The chief cells elaborate pepsinogen, important protein-degrading enzymes that autoactivate in the lumen when pH is 3.5. The acid-secreting parietal cells and intercalated ECL (histamine-secreting) cells are located in the body of the gland. At and above the neck of the gland (not shown) are the mucus neck and surface epithelial cells.

Fig. 11B, full function of each pathway relies on robustness of the others. Thus, blockade of histamine H_2 receptors by drugs such as cimetidine attenuates secretory responses to cholinergic agonists, and interruption of vagal efferents attenuates responses to histamine [15,17,18].

A key feature of the antral mucosa is the presence of gastrin-secreting G cells and somatostatin-secreting D cells. Only recently has it been appreciated that acidity of the gastric lumen activates the secretion of somatostatin, which in turn inhibits secretion of gastrin. The converse is true: alkaline pH reduces somatostatin secretion, which in turn permits circulating gastrin levels to rise. As discussed below, this relationship is a cornerstone in the physiology of meal-stimulated acid secretion. It is important to note that gastrin receptors (classified as gastrin/cholecystokinin type B receptor [CCK_B]) on the parietal cell are largely trophic; that is, they stimulate growth and development of parietal cells [18,19]. In experimental systems looking at parietal cell function in isolation, gastrin is not a strong agonist of acid secretion. The power of gastrin as a secretory agonist lies in its stimulation of histamine release by the ECL cell [17,18]. Fig. 12 summarizes pharmacologic and surgical approaches to inhibition of acid secretion, based on the physiologic concepts outlined in Fig. 11B.

Three endogenous classes of inhibitory neurohumoral signals are somatostatin, epidermal growth factor and transforming growth factor alpha (EGF/TGFα), and prostaglandins of the E and I series. Somatostatin indirectly regulates acid secretion through its effects on gastrin secretion and independent suppression of histamine release from the ECL cell. It remains unclear whether somatostatin directly alters parietal cell responses to secretory stimulation by cholinergic agonists or histamine. Inhibition of acid

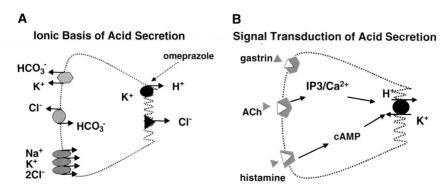

Fig. 11. (*A*) The ionic basis of HC1 secretion includes the H^+/K^+ adenosine triphosphatase (ATPase) localized in the apical membrane of the parietel cell, which is sensitive to inhibition by substituted benzimidazoles such as omeprazole. The movement of Cl^- ions accompanies the luminal secretion of H^+ to maintain electroneutrality. Within the parietal cell, stimulation of acid secretion leads to depletion of intracellular Cl^- amd accumulation of HCO_3^- ions. To address these imbalances, three parallel mechanisms are present in the basolateral membrane: (1) a constitutively active Cl^-/HC_3^- exchanger (identified as anion exchanger isoform AE2); (2) An HCO_3^--independent Cl^- uptake mechanism, the NA^+-K^+-$2Cl^-$ cotransporter (identified as isoform NKCC1); and (3) a Cl^--independent HCO_3^- extrusion mechanism, possibly dependent on NA^+ or K^+, or both. (*B*) Signal transduction pathways related to acid secretion include cholingeric activation of inositol triphosphate release (IP_3), which in turn induces release of Ca^{2+} from intracellular stores in the endoplasmic reticulum. Targets of intracellular Ca^{2+} include calmodulin, a key cofactor in membrane fusion of tubulovesicles with the apical membrane. In addition, release of Ca^{2+} amplifies mitochondrial respiration and ATP production. Histamine released by ECL cells interacts with the H2 receptor to activate adenylyl cyclase, which increases cyclic 3′,5′ adenosine monophosphate (AMP) levels. Interactions of cyclic 3′,5′ adenosine monophosphate (cAMP) and protein kinase A lead to a sequence of events that result in membrane fusion and activation of acid secretion. Both pathways are required for full expression of acid secretion capacity.

secretion by EGF/TGFα occurs within the parietal cell, through modulation of intracellular tyrosine kinase pathways that have downstream regulatory influences on signaling pathways discussed above [14]. Prostaglandin E_2 has effects at several levels, including release of histamine and suppression of intracellular signaling pathways in the parietal cells that are activated by cholinergic agonists and histamine [20,21]. Thus, acid secretion may be inhibited physiologically, by endogenous neurohumoral agents that act at the level of the brain and central nervous system (CNS), at the level of the histamine-secreting ECL cell, and at the level of the parietal cell. Thus far, none of these endogenous inhibitory pathways has provided a basis for clinical interventions in controlling acid secretion.

Alkaline secretion by gastric mucosa

The non-acid secreting mucosa of the gastric antrum and pylorus is characterized by the presence of relatively simple glands populated by mucus- and HCO_3^--secreting surface epithelium. The surface epithelium, in

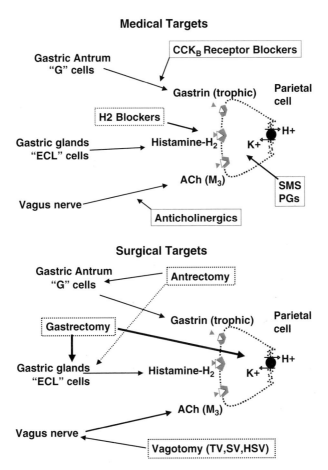

Fig. 12. Pharmacologic approaches to control of acid secretion include targeting of individual receptors that modulate acid secretion or that influence secretion of the paracrine hormone histamine by the ECL cell. Surgical approaches remove the organs (gastric antrum, corpus) or interrupt the stimulatory neurologic pathways (abdominal vagus nerves). Medical and surgical approaches rely on primary effects as well as secondary disabling of other pathways of stimulation.

both the antrum and the corpus/fundus regions, is the basis of the "mucosal barrier." The mechanisms thought to protect the mucosa from back-flux of H^+ from the lumen are illustrated in Fig. 13.

Gastric digestion and contributions to downstream absorption

The stomach contributes to digestion of solid food by mixing chyme with acid and pepsin (pepsinogen autoactivated in the presence of luminal acid), which helps break down protein to simple peptides that will be absorbed or broken down further by intestinal peptidases. Subpopulations of parietal

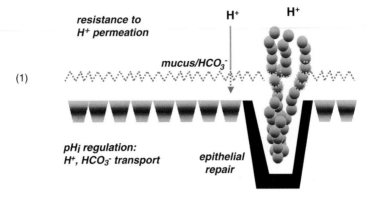

resistance to
H⁺ permeation

H⁺   **H⁺**

mucus/HCO₃⁻

(1)

pHᵢ regulation:
H⁺, HCO₃⁻ transport   *epithelial*
repair

Mucosal blood flow

Fig. 13. Much research has focused on protection against H⁺ back-diffusion. Mechanisms include the mucus-bicarbonate gel and the intrinsic resistance of the surface epithelium to H⁺ diffusion, which is a property of the apical membranes and tight junctions, and possibly related to surface phospholipid composition. An important property of gastric mucus is its ability to retard diffusion of H⁺ not just from the lumen, but from the side; that is, as it bubbles up from the mouth of the gastric gland. Located in the basolateral membranes of the surface epithelial cells are mechanisms promoting HCO₃ accumulation and H⁺ extrusion. When the mucosa is injured by normal abrasion with chyme or by exposure to topical irritants such as aspirin or ethanol, re-epithelialization of the surface occurs quickly, a process known as mucosal restitution. Persistent conditions of injury lead to acceleration of intrinsic processes of repair, and may also require redistribution of blood flow and increases in mucosal perfusion.

cells also secrete intrinsic factor, an essential cofactor in the absorption of vitamin B_{12} downstream in the terminal ileum. Gastric acid itself enables absorption of specific metals and nonmetal cations, including Ca^{2+}, Fe^{3+}, and other trace metals. At low pH, Ca^{2+} is more fully released from binding bases, and is thus more available for absorption in the duodenum. Similarly, Fe^{2+} auto-oxidizes in the presence of luminal acid, placing it in a form more easily absorbed in the small intestine.

Gastric motility

The stomach has three layers of muscularis: an inner circular layer, a middle longitudinal layer, and an outer but incomplete oblique layer. Motor functions in the stomach are segregated by region. The fundus relaxes as fluids and solids enter the esophagus, a response known as receptive relaxation, and further as food actually enters the funds, a process known as adaptive relaxation [22,23]. This response allows the liquid to pool in the fundic pouch while the solid components of the meal remain in the mainstream of flow toward the pylorus.

On the greater curvature, in muscularis of the upper corpus, lies the primary electrical pacemaker of the stomach. Superimposed on the basic electrical rhythm of the pacemaker, the corpus and antrum engage in a coordinated propulsion of the luminal contents toward the pylorus. The pylorus itself acts as a sieve, remaining open in anticipation of the wave of peristalsis. As the wave advances, small particles pass through the pyloric sphincter; when the wave hits, the pylorus closes, thereby acting as a barricade. The chyme, propelled with increasing velocity against the pyloric sphincter, is thus broken up by enzymatic digestion in combination with mechanical disruption.

Satiety

The role of the stomach in regulating food intake has become an increasingly important theme, especially with increasing numbers of procedures for bariatric surgery. In this regard, the recently described hormone ghrelin has assumed central importance. Ghrelin is an appetite-stimulating hormone that is released by gastric mucosal to the portal circulation when the stomach is empty, passing to the central circulation to stimulate appetite centers in the hypothalamus; circulating levels of ghrelin fall precipitously as soon as the stomach begins to fill. In bariatric surgical procedures that create small pouches that distend quickly, baseline and premeal peaks of ghrelin are suppressed, suggesting that blunting of ghrelin responses may contribute to suppression of appetite after bariatric surgery. By no means is ghrelin the dominant signal for control of satiety (Fig. 14) [24], but its effects must be understood in the context of other neural and hormonal inputs to satiety centers in the pituitary.

An integrated view of gastric function in response to a meal

When chyme, containing both liquid and sold components, enters the stomach, the process of true digestion begins, distinguished from mastication upstream in the oral cavity and absorption that occurs downstream in the intestine. Between meals, gastric secretion in the average adult is relatively low, producing an average of 4 mEq/hr ($\sim$25 mL of pure gastric juice). The sensation if hunger is mediated by a multidimensional process, including conditioned behaviors [25] and release of key hormones such as ghrelin. The sight and smell of food initiates the vagally-mediated, Pavlovian response, which not only activates salivation in the oral cavity but also initiates the cephalic phase of acid secretion in the stomach. In addition, gastrin-releasing peptide (GRP) is released by vagal inputs to antral G-cells, thereby activating early release of gastrin in anticipation of the passage of the meal to the stomach. About 15% of the total quantity of acid that is secreted in response to a meal [16] is attributed to the cephalic phase. The capacity to secrete acid given only the sight, smell, and chewing of food leads to a reasonably reliable method for monitoring the completeness of vagotomy in postoperative patients. In one study, Bradshaw and Thirlby [26] used such sham-feeding protocols to identify patients with unexpectedly

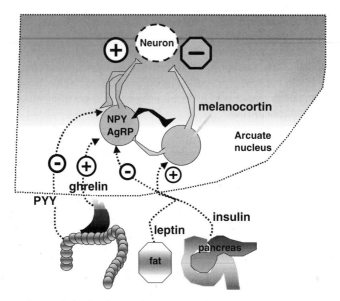

Fig. 14. Neurohumoral circuits that regulate satiety. Effector neurons (*top*) regulate eating and energy expenditure. At the next level, two sets of neurons in the arcuate nucleus excite neuropeptide Y (NPY)/nucleus agouti related protein (AgRP) or inhibit (melanocortin) the effector neurons. At the peripheral level, hormones such as insulin and leptin stimulate melanocortin-secreting neurons and inhibit NPY/AgRP neurons, thereby attenuating the desire for eating. Peptide YY (PYY), secreted from the colon in response to feeding, is inhibitory to feeding, whereas ghrelin, acting on NPY/AgRP neurons, is excitatory to eating. (*Adapted from* Schwartz MW, Morton GJ. Obesity: Keeping hunger at bay. Nature 2002;418:596; with permission.)

robust vagal responses to a meal, thereby identifying those patients as candidates for additional antisecretory therapy after vagotomy.

In addition to stimulation of acid secretion, the cephalic phase of vagal stimulation also prepares the gastric fundus to relax in anticipation of the flow of chyme into the stomach [22]. The predigestive phase of acid secretion is mediated by cholinergic efferents, but the process of receptive relaxation is mediated by noncholinergic vagal fibers, involving capsaicin-sensitive fibers that elaborate calcitonin gene related peptide (CGRP) and nitric oxide (NO) as neurotransmitters [23].

Food entering the gastric lumen initially segregates into solid components that, by and large, stay within the mainstream, and liquid components that are diverted to the expanding gastric fundus (adaptive relaxation). Distension of the gastric antrum and increases in pressure stimulate peristalsis and churning within the mainstream of the gastric lumen, a process known as trituration. The admixture of acid, activation of pepsinogen, and the increasingly accessible protein components of the chyme leads to rapid breakdown into smaller peptides. Expansion of the intragastric space, increase in luminal pressure, the appearance of small peptides, and the rapid buffering of luminal acid all lead to suppression of somatostatin secretion and enhancement of gastrin release, which in turn activates local release of histamine from ECL cells. Local vagally mediated reflexes enhance parietal cell responsiveness to histamine. This gastric phase of acid secretion is responsible for about 75% of the total secretory response [16]. In normal subjects, the integrated secretory response to a steak meal is about 90 to 100 mEq over 3.5 hours, equivalent to approximately 650 to 700 cc of gastric juice [16].

Importantly, during this period, trituration of chyme leads to its pulverization and accumulation of small fragments that will pass through the sieve created by the pylorus just before the advancing wave of peristalsis. As the lumen contracts, sequestered liquid from the fundus starts to pass into the mainstream and facilitates a more thorough mixing of the remnants of the chyme with pepsins.

Potentially important physiologic disturbances of mixing and motility occur in response to vagotomy, which is usually accompanied by loss of the pyloric gating function. These consequences include: (1) early emptying of liquids, caused by loss of receptive and adaptive relaxation, which leads to bloating and gas pain even in the absence of pyloric obstruction [27,28]; (2) rapid emptying of hyperosmotic or inadequately digested chyme into the intestine, caused by bypass of loss of pyloric function, which leads to early and late dumping syndromes [27,29]; and (3) bile backwash and overgrowth of bacteria in the normally clean (<100 cfu/ml) gastric lumen caused by loss of gastric acidity, which leads to disturbances in mucosal proliferation and growth and perhaps malignant transformation [30,31]. These predictable disturbances should be monitored and taken into account in assessment of the efficacy and risks of emerging bariatric procedures.

Evolving areas of interest in gastric physiology

Despite intense interest over 200 years, there remains no satisfactory answer to the question posed by William Beaumont [32]: why does the stomach not digest itself? Whereas the last 200 years of inquiry have been directed at understanding conditions and mechanisms of acid secretion, new interventions and procedures may be expected to challenge our understanding of the mucosal resistance to the damaging effects of luminal acid and other hostile luminal conditions. Over the years, several paradoxes have been presented by experimental work in each of the putative dimensions of gastroprotection. For example, considerable interest attended observations that physical properties of gastric mucus are altered by ambient pH [33]. Extracted from the interface of the gastric mucosa and lumen, mucin resists bulk flow of acid but not diffusion of protons [34]. Gastric mucin is a complex structure, characterized by cysteine-rich clusters and noncovalent binding of protein, lipid, and carbohydrate components [35,36]. Mucin components are also thought to play a role in mucosal proliferation, growth, and renewal [37], identifying them as putative growth factors that might contribute to healing of chronic peptic ulcers [38] and pathogenesis of malignancy [39].

Equally intriguing are recent observations that the interaction between food and bacteria in the upper gastrointestinal (GI) tract profoundly influence mucosal function, even under physiologic conditions. Recent studies have suggested that dietary nitrate (NO_3^-, found in many meats and foodstuffs) are rapidly reduced to nitrite (NO_2^-) by nitrate reductase systems of commensal bacteria that reside in the oropharynx [40,41]. These nitrites are converted by gastric acid to nitric oxide [42], a highly consequential and biologically active agent that influences gastric mucosal function, motility, and blood flow. Depending on the circumstances, NO and its breakdown products may be considered helpful or harmful to mucosal function and integrity [43–45]. In recent studies, it has been suggested that therapeutic manipulations affecting function of the foregut (oral cavity to duodenum) may alter mucosal function, growth, and barrier function at the gastro-esophageal junction, an area increasingly recognized for its susceptibility to metaplasia and malignant transformation [46]. These considerations emphasize that surgeons should be at the forefront of investigation into biochemical and physiological stresses that might be caused by emerging pharmacologic interventions and invasive procedures (surgical, minimally invasive, or endoscopic) of the stomach and GE junction.

References

[1] Baron JH. The discovery of gastric acid. Gastroenterology 1979;76:1056–74.
[2] Rosenfeld L. The last alchemist—the first biochemist: J.B. van Helmont (1577–1644). Clin Chem 1985;31:1755–60.
[3] Modlin IM. From Prout to the proton pump: a history of the science of gastric acid secretion and the surgery of peptic ulcer. Surg Gynecol Obstet 1990;170:81–96.
[4] Rosenfeld L. William Prout: early 19th century physician chemist. Clin Chem 2003;49:699–705.
[5] Osler WS. William Beaumont. A pioneer American physiologist. JAMA 1902;39:1223–31.
[6] Code CF, Higgins JA, Moll JC, et al. The influence of acid on the gastric absorption of water, sodium and potassium. Journal of Physiology 1963;166:110–9.
[7] Davenport HW, Warner HA, Code CF. Functional significance of gastric mucosal barrier to sodium. Gastroenterology 1964;47:142–52.
[8] Feldman M, Cryer B, McArthur KE, et al. Effects of aging and gastritis on gastric acid and pepsin secretion in humans: a prospective study. Gastroenterology 1996;110:1043–52.
[9] Hurwitz A, Brady DA, Schaal SE, et al. Gastric acidity in older adults. JAMA 1997;278:659–62.
[10] Jaszewski R, Ehrinpreis MN, Majumdar APN. Aging and cancer of the stomach and colon. Front Biosci 1999;4:322–8.
[11] Oi M, Oshida K, Sugimura S. The location of gastric ulcer. Gastroenterology 1968;54(Suppl):740–1.
[12] Jackson RG. Anatomy of the vagus nerves in the region of the lower esophagus and the stomach. Anatomic Record 1949;103:1–18.
[13] Kajitani T. The general rules for the gastric cancer study in surgery and pathology. Part I. Clinical classification. Jpn J Surg 1981;11:127–39.

[14] Yao X, Forte JG. Cell biology of acid secretion by the parietal cell. Annu Rev Physiol 2003; 65:103–31.
[15] Samuelson LC, Hinkle KL. Insights into the regulation of gastric acid secretion through analysis of genetically engineered mice. Annu Rev Physiol 2003;65:383–400.
[16] Goldschmiedt M, Feldman M. Gastric secretion in health and disease. In: Sleisenger MH, Fordtran JS, editors. Gastrointestinal diseases. 5th edition. Philadelphia: W.B. Saunders Co; 1993. p. 524–44.
[17] Sanders MJ, Soll AH. Characterization of receptors regulating secretory function in the fundic mucosa. Annu Rev Physiol 1986;48:89–101.
[18] Schubert ML. Gastric secretion. Curr Opin Gastroenterol 2003;19:519–25.
[19] Huang Y, Tola VB, Fang P, et al. Partitioning of aquaporin-4 water channel mRNA and protein in gastric glands. Dig Dis Sci 2003;48:2027–36.
[20] Nylander O, Berglindh T, Obrink KJ. Prostaglandin interaction with histamine release and parietal cell activity in isolated gastric glands. Am J Physiol 1986;250:G607–16.
[21] Choquet A, Magous R, Bali JP. Gastric mucosal endogenous prostanoids are involved in the cellular regulation of acid secretion from isolated parietal cells. J Pharmacol Exp Ther 1993; 266:1306–11.
[22] Jahnberg T, Abrahamsson H, Jansson G, et al. Vagal gastric relaxation in the dog. Scand J Gastroenterol 1977;12:221–4.
[23] Arakawa T, Uno H, Fukuda T, et al. New aspects of gastric adaptive relaxation, reflex after food intake for more food: involvement of capsaicin-sensitive sensory nerves and nitric oxide. J Smooth Muscle Res 1997;33:81–8.
[24] Schwartz MW, Morton GJ. Obesity: keeping hunger at bay. Nature 2002;418:595–7.
[25] Pavlov I. Lectures on conditioned reflexes: twenty-five years of objective study of the higher nervous activity (behaviour) of animals. New York: International Publishers; 1928.
[26] Bradshaw BG, Thirlby RC. The value of sham-feeding tests in patients with postgastrectomy syndromes. Arch Surg 1993;128:982–6.
[27] Soybel DI, Zinner MJ. Complications following gastric operations. In: Zinner MJ, editor. Maingot's abdominal operations. 9th edition. Stamford (CT): Appleton & Lange; 1997. p. 1029–56.
[28] Le Blanc-Louvry I, Savoye G, Maillot C, et al. An impaired accommodation of the proximal stomach to a meal is associated with symptoms after distal gastrectomy. Am J Gastroenterol 2003;98:2642–7.
[29] Hasler WL. Dumping syndrome. Curr Treat Options Gastroenterol 2002;5:139–45.
[30] Kubo M, Sasako M, Gotoda T, et al. Endoscopic evaluation of the remnant stomach after gastrectomy: proposal for a new classification. Gastric Cancer 2002;5:83–9.
[31] Johannesson KA, Hammar E, Stael von Holstein C. Mucosal changes in the gastric remnant: long-term effects of bile reflux diversion and Helicobacter pylori infection. Eur J Gastroenterol Hepatol 2003;15:35–40.
[32] Beaumont W, Osler WS. Experiments and observations on the gastric juice and the physiology of digestion: William Beaumont. Together with a biographical essay, "William Beaumont: a pioneer American physiologist," by Sir William Osler. Mineola (NY): Dover; 1959.
[33] Bhaskar KR, Garik P, Turner BS, et al. Viscous fingering of HCl through gastric mucin. Nature 1992;360:458–61.
[34] Phillipson M. Acid transport through gastric mucus. Ups J Med Sci 2004;109:1–24.
[35] Bhaskar KR, Gong DH, Bansil R, et al. Profound increase in viscosity and aggregation of pig gastric mucin at low pH. Am J Physiol 1991;261:G827–32.
[36] Gong DH, Turner B, Bhaskar KR, et al. Lipid binding to gastric mucin: protective effect against oxygen radicals. Am J Physiol 1990;259:G681–6.
[37] Taupin D, Podolsky DK. Trefoil factors: initiators of mucosal healing. Nat Rev Mol Cell Biol 2003;4:721–32.

[38] Farrell JJ, Taupin D, Koh TJ, et al. TFF2/SP-deficient mice show decreased gastric proliferation, increased acid secretion, and increased susceptibility to NSAID injury. J Clin Invest 2002;109:193–204.

[39] Wang TC, Goldenring JR. Inflammation intersection: gp130 balances gut irritation and stomach cancer. Nat Med 2002;8:1080–2.

[40] Gladwin MT. Haldane, hot dogs, halitosis, and hypoxic vasodilation: the emerging biology of the nitrite anion. J Clin Invest 2004;113:19–21.

[41] Bjorne HH, Petersson J, Phillipson M, et al. Nitrite in saliva increases gastric mucosal blood flow and mucus thickness. J Clin Invest 2004;113:106–14.

[42] Benjamin N, O'Driscoll F, Dougall H, et al. Stomach NO synthesis. Nature 1994;368:502.

[43] West SD, Mercer DW. Bombesin-induced gastroprotection. Ann Surg 2005;241:227–31.

[44] Halliwell B, Zhao K, Whiteman M. Nitric oxide and peroxynitrite. The ugly, the uglier and the not so good: a personal view of recent controversies. Free Radic Res 1999;31:651–69.

[45] Fiorucci S, Santucci L, Wallace JL, et al. Interaction of a selective cyclooxygenase-2 inhibitor with aspirin and NO-releasing aspirin in the human gastric mucosa. Proc Natl Acad Sci U S A 2003;100:10937–41.

[46] McColl KE. When saliva meets acid: chemical warfare at the oesophagogastric junction. Gut 2005;54:1–3.

ELSEVIER
SAUNDERS

SURGICAL
CLINICS OF
NORTH AMERICA

Surg Clin N Am 85 (2005) 895–906

Medical Management of Acid-Peptic Disorders of the Stomach

Sheila Eswaran, MD, Michael A. Roy, MD*

*Portland Gastroenterology Associates, 1200 Congress Street,
Suite 300 Portland, ME 04102-2129, USA*

As a physiologic milieu, there is none so inhospitable as the human stomach. Over the course of a lifetime, the gastric epithelium is at all times responsible for maintaining a pH gradient of 10^6 without itself being auto-digested. In addition to withstanding such a withering onslaught of hydrogen ions, the stomach must also defend itself against other noxious endogenous agents such as pepsin, bile, and pancreatic enzymes. As a consequence of nonphysiologic events, the gastric mucosa may also be attacked by exogenous agents such as alcohol or aspirin and other nonsteroidal anti-inflammatory drugs (NSAIDs).

Historically, medical therapy of acid-peptic disorders of the stomach focused primarily on counteracting the effects of acid secretion. Thus, the simple addition of various alkali in an effort to titrate gastric hydrochloric acid was the mainstay of therapy for decades. As the physiology of gastric acid secretion was elucidated, the advent of antisecretory therapy arrived in the 1970s. Further understanding of the nature of the gastric mucosal barrier led to a handful of therapies designed to enhance or protect the latter. Finally, the pivotal role of *Helicobacter pylori* as the causative agent of type B chronic gastritis and most peptic ulcer disease has led to a paradigm shift in our understanding and treatment of these disorders.

Following a description of the relevant physiology and biochemistry of gastric acid secretion and the gastric mucosal barrier, this article describes the current medicinal arsenal available to treat acid-peptic disorders of the stomach.

---

* Corresponding author.
E-mail address: Roym@mmc.org (M.A. Roy).

0039-6109/05/$ - see front matter © 2005 Elsevier Inc. All rights reserved.
doi:10.1016/j.suc.2005.05.006   *surgical.theclinics.com*

Physiology of gastric acid secretion and the gastric mucosal barrier

Acid-peptic disorders are generally considered to result from an imbalance between noxious agents and the gastroduodenal mucosa's innate defense mechanisms. Ever since the unique, pioneering studies of William Beaumont, hydrochloric acid and pepsin have been recognized as the predominant intrinsic harmful agents to the gastroduodenal mucosa. During the latter half of the twentieth century, H pylori and nonsteroidal anti-inflammatory drugs (NSAIDs) have been identified as the leading extrinsic causes of peptic ulcer disease.

Chief cells secrete pepsinogen, the precursor of pepsin, and hydrochloric acid is secreted by parietal cells (Table 1). Multiple neural and hormonal mediators stimulate and inhibit the release of these gastric secretions. Oxyntic glands in the fundus and body of the stomach contain mucous glands, chief cells, parietal cells, histamine-secreting enterochromaffin-like (ECL) cells and somatostatin-secreting D cells. Somatostatin is the primary inhibitory hormone. Mucous cells, gastrin (G) cells, D cells, and chief cells make up the pyloric glands located in the antrum and pylorus [1,2].

Gastric acid secretion is stimulated by the presence of food at different phases of digestion. The cephalic phase represents the activation of the vagus nerve to release the neurotransmitter acetylcholine, triggered by the sight, smell, and taste of food. As food enters the stomach, the gastric phase begins and amino acids trigger the release of gastrin from gastric cells. During the intestinal phase, intestinal distention, and presence of amino acids, carbohydrates, and lipids activate acid secretion.

Parietal cells release hydrochloric acid in response to gastrin, acetylcholine (M3 receptor) and histamine (H2 receptor). Intracellularly, gastrin and acetylcholine activate the phosphoinositide-calcium cascade, whereas histamine activates cyclic adenosine monophosphate (cAMP) cascade. Both of these pathways lead to the production of ATP, which is the substrate for the luminal H^+, K^+-ATPase pump (Fig. 1).

Table 1
Gastric mucosal cells and secretions

Gland	Cells	Secretion
Oxyntic gland	Chief cells	Pepsinogen
	Parietal cells	Hydrochloric acid
	D cells	Somatostatin
	Mucous epithelial cells	Mucus + bicarbonate
	ECL cells	Histamine
Pyloric gland	Chief cells	Pepsinogen
	D cells	Somatostatin
	Mucous epithelial cells	Mucous + bicarbonate
	G cells	Gastrin

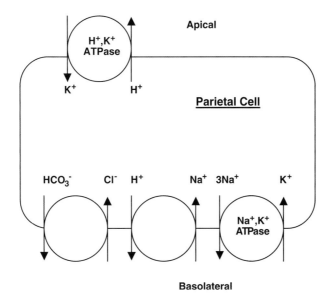

Fig. 1. Parietal cell H^+, K^+-ATPase.

Chief cells (peptic cells) release pepsinogen in response to acetylcholine and histamine. The acidic gastric environment converts pepsinogen to pepsin, which causes protein breakdown and may contribute to mucosal injury.

The discovery of *H pylori* has redefined our understanding of acid-peptic disorders. The organism may be transmitted person-to-person through fecal-oral or oral-oral routes, and is recognized as the primary factor in predisposing patients to chronic type B gastritis and peptic ulcer disease. *H pylori* is uniquely adapted to life in human stomach, living in the relatively neutral microenvironment of the gastric mucous layer attached to gastric epithelial cells. Endowed with a highly active urease, the organism is able to further buffer the acidity of its immediate environment by converting host urea into ammonium ion and carbon dioxide. This feature of *H pylori* has been exploited clinically for various diagnostic tests.

H pylori's pathogenicity is mediated by various toxins, as well as by host immune response to the organism. Differences exist between different strains of *H pylori*. All strains contain the gene for cytotoxin VacA, which causes severe tissue damage and facilitates transport of urea to the epithelium. An associated gene, CagA, coexpresses the VacA gene in some. Bacteria that express both genes are associated with a higher frequency of ulcers and premalignant lesions [3].

NSAIDs are the second most common trigger for the development of peptic ulcers. NSAIDs injure the gastrointestinal mucosa by direct topical damage, and by decreasing prostaglandin synthesis systemically and at the mucosal level [4]. Epidemiologically, the importance of NSAIDs as a cause of gastric disease is eclipsing that of *H pylori* as the latter wanes in prevalence in the industrialized world.

Gastric and duodenal defense mechanisms are in place to prevent and repair injury to the mucosa. This defense is divided into pre-epithelial, epithelial, and postepithelial mechanisms, although the process is dynamic. The mucous-bicarbonate layer composes the pre-epithelial barrier by maintaining a neutral environment (pH 7) in the presence of highly acidic (pH 2) lumen contents. Bicarbonate and mucous are secreted by surface epithelium of the gastric and duodenal mucosa. Mucous is 95% water in addition to glycoproteins, which neutralize diffusing hydrogen ions and completely block pepsin passage. A phospholipids component is also present, which creates a hydrophobic layer to repel acid.

Epithelial cells maintain tight junctions between adjacent cells to prevent the entry of caustic agents through the mucosal layer. During superficial injury, a rapid migration of epithelial cells blocks the secretion of acid. This process is termed mucosal restitution. In addition, a mucoid cap made up of mucous, fibrin, and epithelial cells forms with deeper destruction to prevent acid contact with the intracellular matrix. If acid penetrates the early barriers, intracellular Na^+/H^+, Cl^-/HCO_3^- exchangers and Na^+/HCO_3^- cotransporters regulate pH.

Efficient gastric epithelial cell regeneration is regulated by growth factors and prostaglandins. Prostaglandins are naturally occurring 20-carbon chain unsaturated fatty acids. In the gastrointestinal tract, prostaglandin E2 (PGE2) and PGF2 are released by mucosal cells and are said to exert "cytoprotective" effects on the gastroduodenal mucosa. These effects are mediated in part by prostaglandin influences on gastric mucosal bicarbonate and mucous secretion. In addition to the cytoprotective effect of pro-staglandins, there exists a less potent antisecretory effect by inhibiting the effects of histamine-induced cyclic-AMP activation in parietal cells.

The postepithelial defense mechanism relies on adequate mucosal blood flow transporting bicarbonate to surface epithelium for the mucous-bicarbonate barrier. This alkaline tide also protects the lamina propria from acid-peptic injury [5]. Mucosal blood flow is also influenced by local prostaglandin synthesis.

Antisecretory therapy

Anti-cholinergic agents

Anticholinergic drugs affect the parietal cell by inhibiting basal and meal-stimulated gastric acid secretion. Atropine, and to a lesser degree pirenzepine, have systemic side effects such as blurred vision, urinary retention, and dry mouth. Anticholinergic medications such as atropine and pirenzepine have no significant role in peptic ulcer treatment. Other medications, including proton pump inhibitors and histamine-2 receptor blockers, are much more effective and have fewer side effects.

Histamine-2 receptor antagonists

Histamine-2 receptor antagonists have an aromatic ring with a flexible side chain similar to the histamine molecule. These agents bind to the histamine-2 (H2) receptor on the parietal cell to reversibly inhibit the 90% basal and meal-stimulated gastric acid secretion. Research shows H2 receptor antagonists are moderately effective, healing 70% to 80% of duodenal ulcers and 55% to 65% of gastric ulcers in 4 to 6 weeks.

H2 receptor antagonists are available by prescription and over the counter. Currently available H2 receptor antagonists include cimetidine, ranitidine, famotidine, and nizatidine. Dosing for active ulcers is twice a day for 4 to 8 weeks. H2 receptor blockers can be used once before bed for maintenance therapy, although tachyphylaxis occurs frequently with chronic administration. Absorption is not affected by the ingestion of food, but is decreased by antacids and sucralfate. Peak blood level occurs in 1 to 3 hours. Oral cimetidine, ranitidine, and famotidine are metabolized by the first-pass mechanism in the liver. Oral nizatidine and all intravenous preparations have a 100% bioavailability and are not metabolized by the liver first pass. Hepatic metabolites are excreted by the kidney. There is no indication for dose adjustment in hepatic dysfunction, but renal dosing is necessary with a reduced creatinine clearance. All H2 receptor antagonists are categorized by the Food and Drug Administration (FDA) as class B agents in pregnancy.

Other medications that rely on an acidic environment to be absorbed should be used with caution. Ketoconazole and ampicillin may have decreased serum concentrations and bioavailability. In addition, cimetidine, and to a lesser degree ranitidine, bind to the enzyme cytochrome P450 and inhibit Phase I oxidation and dealkalylation, increasing the serum concentrations of drugs that depend on this enzyme for metabolism (Table 2) [6]. Famotidine and nizatidine do not affect CYP450.

All H2 receptor antagonists have a similar side effect profile. Adverse effects occur less than 4% in most studies. Cimetidine was the first of the class and therefore has been studied the most. Cimetidine, when given chronically or at higher doses, has an anti-androgenic effect manifested by gynecomastia and impotence. These side effects are reversible after discontinuation of the drug. Myelosuppression, leukopenia, neutropenia, anemia, thrombocytopenia, and pancytopenia have been associated with all H2 receptor antagonists. Central nervous system (CNS) side effects such as headache, lethargy, dizziness, depression, memory loss, agitation, confusion, psychosis, and hallucinations can occur, but are more commonly seen in patients who receive intravenous dosing and are elderly, or in those who

Table 2
Significant cytochrome P-450 drug interactions

Enzyme	Drug	Interactions
Cytochrome 3A4	Lansoprazole	Warfarin (minor)
	Clarithromycin	Astemizole, carbamazepine, cisapride, cyclosporine, HMG-CoA reductase inhibitors, indinavir, quinidine, tacrolimus, warfarin
	Omeprazole	Warfarin
	Metronidazole	Cisapride, quinidine
	Cimetidine	Fentanyl, lidocaine, midazolam, nifedipine, quinidine, triazolam, verapamil
Cytochrome 2D6	Cimetidine	Meperidine, propafenone, tricyclic antidepressants
	Clarithromycin	Fluoxetine
Cytochrome 1A2	Cimetidine	Tacrine, theophylline, warfarin
	Clarithromycin	Theopylline
Cytochrome 2C	Cimetidine	Phenytoin
	Omeprazole	Diazepam, phenytoin

Adapted from Michalets EL. Reviews of therapeutics. Update: clinically significant cytochrome P-450 drug interactions. Pharmacotherapy 1998;18(1):84–112.

have renal or hepatic impairment. Although important to consider in patients who have mental status changes, CNS side effects are somewhat uncommon, occurring in fewer than 1% of patients. There may be elevations (two to three times) in hepatic transaminases or mild increases in creatinine, both of which have little clinical significance. There have been case reports of acute hepatitis, but none of renal failure [7].

Proton pump inhibitors

As a class, these drugs bind to the alpha chain on the H^+, K^+-ATPase pump to irreversibly inactivate the enzyme. Proton pump inhibitors (PPIs) act only on actively secreting proton pumps. During fasting, 5% of pumps are active. At mealtime, proton pump inhibitors are able to affect 60% to 70% of H^+, K^+-ATPase pumps. Every 72 hours, new proton pumps are synthesized. PPIs should be given immediately before a meal daily to maximally block both basal and meal-stimulated acid secretion [8]. PPIs are activated by an acid environment, but are also very labile, particularly upon exposure to gastric acid. Therefore, these agents are enteric-coated. The absorption of lansoprazole, pantoprazole, and rabeprazole is delayed by food, but not affected by antacids. Peak serum concentration occurs 2 to 5 hours from ingestion. PPIs are metabolized almost completely by the hepatic CYP450 process, and metabolites are eliminated by the kidney. There is no need for dose adjustment in hepatic or renal disease.

PPIs are remarkably effective antisecretory agents. Duodenal ulcers are decreased by 80% to 100%, and gastric ulcers are decreased by 70% to

85%. Currently available PPIs include omeprazole, esomeprazole, lanso-prazole, pantoprazole, and rabeprazole.

Duration of treatment with PPIs is typically 4 to 8 weeks for active peptic ulcer disease. Chronic therapy may be indicated for hypersecretory states or for patients who must continue NSAIDs. Maintenance PPI therapy is more effective than misoprostol or H2 receptor antagonists for NSAID-induced ulcer relapse [9]. Tolerance or tachyphylaxis is not seen as with the H2 receptor antagonists. Sustained therapy commonly leads to hypergastrine-mia caused by the profound degree of acid secretory inhibition achieved. Although seen in early animal studies, the development of gastric carcinoid lesions related to hypergastrinemia has proven to be of theoretical concern only in humans. Recently, concerns have been raised regarding the development of pneumonia in patients on chronic PPI therapy. Other complications of chronic PPI use, such as dietary iron and vitamin B_{12} malabsorption, have been trivial or nonexistent in clinical practice.

Like H2 receptor antagonists, PPIs are well-tolerated by patients. The most common side effects are headaches, diarrhea, abdominal pain, constipation, and nausea. Recent studies also report an increased risk of community-acquired pneumonia in patients on acid suppression [10]. In a given patient who has unacceptable side effects, substituting a different PPI may be well-tolerated. In addition, patients and physicians must be aware of drug-drug interactions. Because PPIs increase intragastric pH, absorption of medications such was ketoconazole and ampicillin will be diminished, and digoxin absorption will be enhanced. Omeprazole also affects the CYP450 enzyme, thereby reducing the clearance of warfarin, diazepam, and phenytoin. With the exception of omeprazole, which is an FDA class C agent, all PPIs are class B agents during pregnancy.

Agents influencing the gastric mucosal barrier

Sucralfate

Sucralfate is sucrose with the 8 hydroxyl groups substituted for by aluminum hydroxide and sulfate. In an acidic environment, the aluminum and sulfate disassociate to form a sulfide. This highly polar anion binds to cations, such as proteins and mucins, to coat mucosal defects. This activity forms a protective barrier and stimulates bicarbonate, mucous, and growth factor release. Sucralfate has generally been underused, in part due to the four-times-a day dosing versus single-dose PPIs. Because only 3% to 5% of sucralfate is absorbed, there are few systemic side effects. In patients who have chronic renal insufficiency, there may be a rise in serum aluminum levels, but toxicity is rare. Aluminum binds to phosphorus, preventing absorption, and may cause hypophosphatemia. Constipation and drug interactions (fluoroquinolones, phenytoin, and warfarin) can occur in some patients. Sucralfate, an FDA class B agent, is safe to use during pregnancy.

Prostaglandin analogs

Misoprostol inhibits gastric acid secretion and stimulates defense mechanisms. This antisecretory activity is less potent than H2 blockers. The reduction of nocturnal, basal, and meal-stimulated acid peaks 30 minutes after ingestion and lasts 90 minutes. Misoprostol is excreted by the kidney, but renal dose adjustments are not necessary. The most common side effects are diarrhea-caused increase motility in the gastrointestinal tract and an increase in electrolyte and water secretion. Misoprostol also causes smooth muscle contraction, specifically uterine smooth muscle. Misoprostol, anFDA class X agent, is an abortifacient and is contraindicated in pregnancy.

Misoprostol is the only FDA-approved prostaglandin analog approved for the prevention of NSAID-induced peptic ulcer disease. The dose of misoprostol is 800 mcg per day in two or four divided doses for 4 weeks. Because of high cost, side effects, and frequent dosing schedule compared with alternative agents, misoprostol is less commonly used (Table 3) [11].

Bismuth compounds

Although bismuth is less widely used for peptic ulcer disease because of the increasing efficacy of other agents, it remains a standard over-the-counter medication for many types of dyspepsia. Bismuth subsalicylate, in a liquid or tablet form, has multiple proposed mechanisms of action. Because of the possible antimicrobial effect, bismuth has been approved for the treatment of *H pylori*. Bismuth also forms a complex with mucin to coat the ulcer, and stimulates the release of bicarbonate and prostaglandin.

Less than 1% percent of bismuth is absorbed. Once in the colon, bacteria convert salicylate to a sulfide, causing black stools. Systemic side effects,

Table 3
Comparison average wholesale price

Medication	Average wholesale price of trade drug (generic price)[a]
Cimetidine 300 mg	1.36 (0.09)
Ranitidine 150 mg	2.30 (1.56)
Famotidine 20 mg	1.97 (1.74)
Nizatidine 150 mg	3.05 (2.38)
Omeprazole 20 mg	4.43 (4.15)
Esomeprazole 20 mg	4.97
Lansoprazole 30 mg	4.96
Pantoprazole 40 mg	3.95
Rabeprazole 20 mg	4.71
Sucralfate 1 gm	1.26 (0.70)
Misoprostol 100 mcg	1.26 (0.82)
Bismuth subsalicylate 120 ml	3.22

[a] In dollars and cents. Actual purchase price will differ.
Data from Cardinal Health. Available at: http://www.cardinal.com/. Accessed April 1, 2005.

such as neurotoxicity, occur rarely when given in high doses for extended periods of time. Bismuth has a class C/D FDA rating during pregnancy.

Other aspects of therapy

Helicobacter pylori

The foundation of peptic ulcer therapy is the eradication of *H pylori*, defined as the absence of the microbe 4 weeks after appropriate antibiotic treatment. Patients who have peptic ulcer disease should be treated for *H pylori* infection unless another cause of the ulcer, such as NSAIDs, is invoked. The identification of *H pylori* by urease breath testing, serology, or culture is not indicated for first-time infections because of cost and low sensitivity, but may have a role in treatment failures or reinfection.

Therapy centers on various combinations of amoxicillin, bismuth, clarithromycin, metronidazole, and PPIs. Combinations have arisen due to antibiotic resistant *H pylori*. Ten to 60% of *H pylori* isolates demonstrate metronidazole resistance. Resistance to clarithromycin and amoxicillin resistance is also seen. In cases of treatment failure due to resistance, a second course of a different combination is indicated. Reinfection and recrudescence are other causes of peptic ulcer reoccurrence. Reinfection of a new strain of *H pylori* occurs as antibiotic treatment selects out more resilient bacteria. Recrudescence, infection of the same strain, is due to incomplete initial cure or a reinfection due to close contact with other persons infected.

The duration of treatment is 10 to 14 days of dual, triple, or quadruple combination of antibiotics (Table 4) [12]. Dual therapy (ie, two antibiotics with a PPI) has an 85% cure rate. Triple therapy includes bismuth subsalicylate (BSS), metronidazole, and tetracycline with a PPI, and has an excellent eradication rate of 94% to 98%. PPIs can be used to flank the traditional 10 to 14 days to increase efficacy and enhance symptom relief. In the cases of treatment failure or known metronidazole resistance, furazolidone, is used. Noncompliance can be related to the complexity of these regimens, and may be alleviated by the copackaging of medications [13], although this generally results in higher treatment costs.

Nonsteroidal anti-inflammatory drugs

Medication cessation is the primary treatment measure for NSAID-induced peptic ulcer disease. Salsalate, nabumetone, and etodolac are NSAIDs that have less potential for causing peptic ulcer disease. Other analgesics such as acetaminophen or narcotics may be implemented as a substitute. NSAIDs should be avoided and *H pylori* testing may be considered if subjects are at high risk for ulcers. High-risk patients are those who have a history of peptic ulcer disease or *H pylori*, those who are older

Table 4
Helicobacter pylori therapy

Combination therapy for *Helicobacter pylori*	Duration
PPI + amoxicillin 1000 mg + clarithromycin 500 mg	Each drug twice daily for 2 weeks
PPI + metronidazole 500 mg + clarithromycin 500 mg	Each drug twice daily for 2 weeks
Bismuth subsalicylate 525 mg four times daily + metronidazole 500 mg twice daily + tetracycline 500 mg four times daily + PPI four times daily	2 weeks
Bismuth subsalicylate 525 mg four times daily + metronidazole 250 mg four times daily + tetracycline 500 mg four times daily + H2 receptor antagonist	2 weeks with H2 receptor blocker continued for 2 weeks further

Data from Howden C, Hunt R. Guidelines for the management of *Helicobacter pylori* infection. Am J Gastroenterol 1998;93:2330–8.

and have comorbidities, or those taking concomitant corticosteroids or anticoagulation. H2 blockers, PPIs, or sucralfate may be used for treatment of NSAID-induced ulcers, and the inciting drug can be discontinued [14].

A difficult situation arises when the NSAID is unable to be substituted, such as in the cases of refractory pain, intolerance to narcotics, or disease processes that require NSAID treatment principally. If NSAIDs must be used in these populations, it is prudent to cotreat while initiating the drug. PPIs are most effective in prophylaxis. H2 blockers, at high doses, are also effective. PPIs and H2 blockers are also central in treatment of active NSAID-induced ulcers while the provocative drug is continued. PPIs have a cure rate of 95% of NSAID-induced ulcers. With ulcers smaller than 5 mm, H2 blockers have been shown to have a similar cure rate. Although misoprostol has little effect on the symptoms, such as dyspepsia, related to peptic ulcer disease, the healing rate is equivalent to that of PPIs. Sucralfate appears to have no role in the treatment of NSAID-induced ulcers if the NSAID is continued. Generally, if a patient is at high risk for peptic ulcer disease, NSAIDs should be avoided. If NSAIDs must be used from the perspective of the patient or clinician, use of a low-risk NSAID or cotreatment with a PPI or misoprostol should be initiated.

Medical therapy of Zollinger-Ellison syndrome and other hypersecretory states

Hypersecretory states such as the Zollinger-Ellison syndrome are characterized by dramatic increases in acid secretion, driven primarily by pathologic elevations in serum gastrin levels. Before the advent of PPIs, medical therapy had little to offer in either the short-term management of the preoperative patient or in the long-term management of inoperable patients. With omeprazole and its related successors, acid secretion can now be effectively controlled in these patients for long periods of time if necessary [15–18]. Intravenous administration of PPIs is also efficacious in the perioperative patient [19].

Summary

In the past 30 years, medicine has witnessed an unprecedented evolution of thought and practice in the management of acid-peptic disorders of the stomach. This evolution has been fueled by major advances in our understanding of the physiology of acid secretion and of the gastric mucosal barrier. The other pivotal development in our developing understanding of these disorders has been the recognition of *H pylori*'s role in the pathophysiology of peptic ulcer disease, chronic gastritis, and even gastric malignancy. As *H pylori* wanes in significance and medicine is faced with the challenges of treating iatrogenic conditions brought on by ulcerogenic anti-inflammatory drugs, this evolution in thought and practice will likely continue.

References

[1] Ivey KJ. Gastric mucosal barrier. Gastroenterology 1971;61(2):247–57.

[2] Sleisenger M, Feldman M, Friedman L, et al. Sleisenger & Fordtran's gastrointestinal and liver disease: pathophysiology, diagnosis, management. 7th edition. Philadelphia: Saunders; 2002. p. 715–81.

[3] Mobley HL. Defining *Helicobacter pylori* as a pathogen: strain heterogeneity and virulence. Am J Med 1996;100(5A):2S–9S.

[4] Wolfe MM, Lichtenstein DR, Singh G. Gastrointestinal toxicity of nonsteroidal antiinflammatory drugs. N Engl J Med 1999;340(24):1888–99.

[5] Yamada T, Alpers D, Kaplowitz N, et al. Textbook of gastroenterology. 4th edition. Philadelphia: Lippincott Williams and Wilkins; 1999. p. 266–307; 1321–76.

[6] Michalets EL. Reviews of therapeutics. Update: clinically significant cytochrome P-450 drug interactions. Pharmacotherapy 1998;18(1):84–112.

[7] Wolfe MM, Sachs G. Acid suppression: optimizing therapy for gastroduodenal ulcer healing, gastroesophageal reflux disease, and stress-related erosive syndrome. Gastroenterology 2000;118(Suppl 1):S9–31.

[8] Lai KC, Lam SK, Chu KM, et al. Lansoprazole for the prevention of recurrences of ulcer complications from long-term low-dose aspirin use. N Engl J Med 2002;346(26):2033–8.

[9] Hawkey CJ, Karrasch JA, Szczepanski L, et al. Omeprazole compared with misoprostal for ulcers associated with non-steroidal anti-inflammatory drugs: omeprazole vs. misoprostol for NSAID-induced ulcer management. (OMNIUM) Study Group. N Engl J Med 1998;338: 727–34.

[10] Laheij RJ, Sturkenboom MC, Hassing RJ, et al. Risk of community-acquired pneumonia and use of gastric acid-suppressive drug. JAMA 2004;292(16):1955–60.

[11] Cardinal Health. Avialable at: http://www.cardinal.com/. Accessed April 1, 2005.

[12] Howden C, Hunt R. Guidelines for the management of *Helicobacter pylori* infection. Am J Gastroenterol 1998;93(12):2330–8.

[13] Rollins G. Consensus guidelines offer more effective management of *Helicobacter pylori*-related disease. Rep Med Guidel Outcomes Res 2000;11(15):1–2, 5.
[14] Schubert ML. Treatment of NSAID-induced gastroduodenal ulcers. Gastroenterology 1990;99(5):1533–5.
[15] Lamers C, Lind T, Moberg S, et al. Omeprazole in Zollinger-Ellison syndrome. N Engl J Med 1984;310:758–61.
[16] Maton P, Vinayek R, Frucht H, et al. Long-term efficacy and safety of omeprazole in patients with Zollinger-Ellison syndrome: a prospective study. Gastroenterology 1989;97:827–36.
[17] Metz D, Soffer E, Forsmark C, et al. Maintenance oral pantoprazole therapy is effective for patients with Zollinger-Ellison syndrome and idiopathic hypersecretion. Am J Gastroenterol 2003;98:301–7.
[18] Hirschowitz B, Simmons J, Mohnen J. Clinical outcome using lansoprazole in acid hypersecretors with and without Zollinger-Ellison syndrome: a 13-year prospective study. Clin Gastroenterol Hepatol 2005;3:39–48.
[19] Vinayek R, Frucht H, London J, et al. Intravenous omprazole in patients with Zollinger-Ellison syndrome undergoing surgery. Gastroenterology 1990;99:10–6.

ELSEVIER
SAUNDERS

SURGICAL
CLINICS OF
NORTH AMERICA

Surg Clin N Am 85 (2005) 907–929

Surgical Management of Ulcer Disease

Ronald F. Martin, MD[a,b,*]

[a]*Department of Surgery, Marshfield Clinic and Saint Joseph's Hospital,
1000 North Oak Avenue, Marshfield, WI 54449, USA*
[b]*University of Vermont, Burlington, VT 05401, USA*

The history of management of ulcer disease is one of the great stories in the history of general surgery. The surgeons who have helped elucidate the anatomy, physiology, biochemistry, and operative management of patients who have ulcers have earned their place in the historical ranks of our discipline. One is hard-pressed to find a vein of surgical thought with such a rich development of understanding of how anatomic and physiological principles can be used to create a myriad of mechanical solutions to functional as well as mechanical problems. For the beginning student of surgery, this history offers an excellent framework for one of the best examples of surgical investigation turned into practice. For the more senior student of surgery, these disorders provide a seemingly endless opportunity to learn and relearn lessons in management of the surgically ill patient. As with any worthy problem, patients who have these disorders give us an opportunity for great reward, and an equally great chance to be humbled.

As is discussed in the article by Drs. Eswaran and Roy elsewhere in this issue, the nonoperative management of ulcer disease, both acid-mediated and nonsteroidal anti-inflammatory drug (NSAID)-mediated, has made tremendous strides in the last 40 years. The net effect of this progress on surgeons is to have shifted the types of operations that we perform from a combination of emergent operations on ill people and an array of nearly elective operations on not-as-ill people, to ones of a more emergent nature upon generally even more ill patients [1,2]. Also, the relative decrease in the need for these types of operations has left our ranks with a declining number of surgeons who have more than a passing familiarity with the practice of these operations. Though the overall demand for these operations has

* Department of Surgery, Marshfield Clinic and Saint Joseph's Hospital, 1000 North Oak Avenue, Marshfield, WI 54449.

E-mail addresses: martin.ronald@marshfieldclinic.org; rfmltc@charter.net

0039-6109/05/$ - see front matter © 2005 Elsevier Inc. All rights reserved.
doi:10.1016/j.suc.2005.05.002   *surgical.theclinics.com*

diminished, it has not vanished. The intent of this article is to provide a review of the rationale for the management of these patients.

The problems

The consequences of ulcer disease can be distilled to a handful of presentations, with pain, perforation, hemorrhage, and obstruction being chief among them. Operative management of patients who have ulcers for the relief of pain has all but disappeared. Patients who have progressive obstructing ulcer lesions are becoming extraordinarily rare as well. The majority of operations that will be performed in the current era will be for perforation or hemorrhage. The true incidence of surgical emergencies is unclear at this time. Reports from the Asian population in the literature suggest that, although the incidence of operation for overall management of ulcer disease may be decreasing, the incidence of emergent operation for ulcer-related problems is actually increasing [3,4]. The literature in the US population is variably reported as to the increase [5] or decrease in need for emergent operation [6,7]. The operations that are discussed in this article are organized by how they address mechanical or functional obstruction, acid suppression, control of hemorrhage, and repair or control of perforation.

Ulcer classification

Gastric ulcers are classified according to their location or colocation with duodenal ulcers. Originally they were classified into three types: Type I ulcers are located along the lesser curve of the stomach, Type II gastric ulcers either concurrently associated with duodenal ulcers or a historical presence of duodenal ulceration, and Type III gastric ulcers are located in the prepyloric position [8]. A fourth classification was added by Csendes and colleagues [9], Type IV, which is located in the vicinity of the esophagogastric junction. Although many classification schemes are less than helpful (with the possible exception of giving the professor of surgery one more avenue of intellectual investigation of his or her trainees), this one may have actual implications, because the middle two types of gastric ulcers are likely to be acid-mediated, and the Type I and Type IV ulcers are more likely to be associated with malignancy. Duodenal ulcers are rarely related to malignancy, and are much more likely to be related to acid-mediated phenomena or NSAID-related ulcer. One caveat that each surgeon should bear in mind is that ulcers located in unusual locations may be indicative of some extraordinary process taking place. For example, ulcers in the third and fourth portion of the duodenum or small bowel not associated with NSAID use may be suggestive of a hypergastrinemic state, such as Zollinger-Ellison syndrome.

Perforation

During the nineteenth century, perforation from ulcer disease was a rare occurrence [10]. The incidence of this problem had markedly increased throughout the twentieth century, peaking for men around the 1950s, though it appears to continue to increase for women. In at least one study from Norway [11], the incidence of perforation for peptic ulcer for men and women was converging as of the 1990s. Multiple explanations for this are offered, including the aging of the population and the increase in the number of persons who smoke cigarettes or take NSAIDs. The two major factors associated with perforation of peptic ulcer are thought to be cigarette smoking and NSAID use; these are thought to contribute to perforation in greater than 75% and 20% to 30% of patients who perforate, respectively [10].

The role of *Helicobacter pylori* in perforation is less clear. A study from Hong Kong [12] showed that 70% of patients who had perforated duodenal ulcer had positive biopsies for *H pylori*. This infection rate was not remarkably different from the 55% prevalence of *H pylori* in the general population. A study from the United Arab Emirates [1] reported 29 patients who underwent simple closure of perforated DU, and were tested for *Helicobacter* by urease breath test on postoperative day 8. Twenty-four of the 29 patients were positive for urease activity. In a report from the United Kingdom [13], 47% of patients who had perforated DU were found to be positive for *Helicobacter* by enzyme linked immunosorbent assay (ELISA). This compared with 50% of the control population, and suggested no relationship between *Helicobacter* and perforation. Despite the unresolved nature of the importance of *Helicobacter* infection in perforation of ulcers, one would be hard-pressed to find compelling evidence that suggest that eradication of the organism in the patients who present with perforation would not be judicious, based upon what we have learned about eradication of *H pylori* and recurrence in the patient who has nonperforating peptic ulcer. The basis for this last observation is chronicled in greater detail in the article by Drs. Eswaran and Roy elsewhere in this issue.

Hemorrhage

Peptic ulcer disease is the most common cause of upper gastrointestinal hemorrhage. Hemorrhage is the most common cause of death in patients who have acid peptic ulcers, and has become the leading indication for operative management in these patients, surpassing intractable pain since the advent of better pharmacologic acid suppression. Duodenal ulcer is the most common site for hemorrhage in patients who have acid peptic disease. The most common site for bleeding duodenal ulcers is on the posterior wall of the duodenal bulb, overlying the gastroduodenal artery. Initial attempts at evaluation and management include adequate resuscitation with prompt performance of esophagogastroduodenoscopy (EGD). Endoscopic means to manage bleeding from these lesions include heater probe, bicap electrocautery, endoscopic injection, laser photo ablation, endoscopic ligation, and placement of hemoclips. Although some have reported good success with endoscopic hemoclip placement for control of arterial hemorrhage [14] the author has not been able to confirm this finding. The use of endoscopic hemoclips, however, may facilitate in the manual localization of the source of bleeding upon entering the intestinal lumen.

The various methods listed all have reasonably high degrees of efficacy in many patients. Proper selection of patients and judicious timing and application of these technologies is considerably more important than the type of energy source used to create hemostasis. A consensus study released by the National Institutes of Health in 1989 [15] reported a preference for the use of heater probe and multipolar electrocautery for use in endoscopic management of ulcer hemorrhage. Furthermore, substantial reductions in recurrent hemorrhage (approximately 70%) for emergent operation (approximately 60%) and mortality rate (approximately 30%) have been demonstrated by meta-analysis evaluating the use of endoscopic means to control ulcer hemorrhage [16]. Endoscopic means have been sufficiently successful to reduce the requirement for emergent operative management to less than 3% of patients.

Operative priorities in the management of gastrointestinal hemorrhage secondary to acid peptic disease are twofold: (1) control of the hemorrhage and continued resuscitation of the patient to alleviate shock, and (2) treatment of the underlying acid peptic disorder. Transpyloric gastro-duodenotomy followed by oversewing of the base of the duodenal ulcer in four quadrants is performed to control the gastroduodenal artery. The gastroduodenal artery may also be ligated in continuity near its origin, in addition to oversewing the ulcer bed itself. The surgeon is then obligated to make a decision regarding what, if any, further therapy should be used. Operations designed to reduce acid secretion include truncal vagotomy (TV), proximal gastric vagotomy (PGV), posterior vagotomy and anterior seromyotomy, and antrectomy and vagotomy. Factors that allow the surgeon to determine the best approach include the status of the patient in terms of hemodynamic stability at the time of operation, associated comorbid factors in the patient's clinical history, the patient's response to prior pharmacological acid suppression, and the collective abilities of the surgeon and surgical team at the time of operation. These procedures are discussed in greater detail later in this article.

The main objective of controlling the hemorrhage must always be held paramount in consideration. Persistent or recurrent hemorrhage following initial therapy is associated with mortality rates ranging from 10% to 44%, depending on response rate to additional therapy [17–19]. The need to address the potential acid-producing state of the patient concurrently seems to be an issue in evolution. In a major surgical text [8], Johnston wrote, "There is one major difference between the operative treatment of hemorrhage from peptic ulcer and the operative treatment of perforation: the use of a definitive ulcer-curing operation is mandatory in patients who have hemorrhage, whereas in patients who have perforation it is optional." A recent review of the randomized trials of operative management of bleeding from ulcers [2] opines in its concluding comments, "With the new approach, surgery, if necessary, should aim at stopping the hemorrhage and not curing the disease." Certainly over the interval between publications of these two papers (1989 to 2000) there has been a marked increase in our understanding of pathogenesis of ulcers and of the mechanism of action of *H pylori*. Though there may be more to these discordant recommendations than this alone. In Ohmann and coworkers' report on surgical treatment of peptic ulcer hemorrhage [2], it is noted that only five randomized trials for the management of bleeding peptic ulcers were found upon searching the literature. Some of these trials also compared operative intervention versus endoscopic management as well. When one wishes to compare randomized, controlled trails for choice of operation for bleeding from peptic ulcers, we are left with only two Class I trials [17,20]. Table 1 includes the results of those trials, along with the results from four uncontrolled trials that compare operative management. The collective recommendations of these studies range from direct management of the bleeding vessel to a "radical" resection approach. In the two controlled trials [17,20], there was a greater incidence of recurrent hemorrhage with minimal operative management (ie, directly vascular suturing plus or minus vagotomy) than was seen with a more aggressive resection of the antrum with reconstruction. The eventual overall mortality of the two groups in each was not significantly different, although the multicenter trial [17] was stopped early because of a significant difference in fatal recurrent hemorrhage in the more conservatively managed (ie, limited operation) group. In the face of the paucity of quality data, we are left with less-than-clear guidance as to which choice is best under the circumstances of an actively bleeding patient for the short term, and we must either await better information to come forth or continue with our best judgment.

The choice of operation for reduction of long-term risk of recurrent hemorrhage is also less than clear. The role of *H pylori* eradication seems to the author more important for the prevention of long-term prevention of recurrent hemorrhage. Two randomized trials [21,22] have shown recurrent hemorrhage of 0% percent with 1-year follow-up after *Helicobacter* eradication. The control groups in these studies had recurrent hemorrhage rates of 33% and 27%. Other studies show a difference in ulcer recurrence rates, although no significantly different hemorrhage recurrence rate [23]. Therefore, the role for definitive acid suppression for long-term eradication of bleeding risk for ulcer in the era of *H pylori* is, at least, in question.

Table 1
Comparison of emergency operations for peptic ulcer bleeding

Study and year	Study type	Population	Sample size (no.)	Operative treatment	Number	Recurrent bleeding (%)	Mortality (%)	Recommendation
Millat, 1993 [20]	Randomized[a]	DU bleeding	60	Gastric resection, BI + ulcer excision	24			
				Gastric resection, BII + ulcer excision	36	3	23	Gastric resection + ulcer excision
Poxon, 1991 [17]	Randomized[a]	PU bleeding	58	Oversewing + vagotomy	58	17	22	
			67	Partial gastrectomy	25			
				Oversewing + vagotomy	35	0	19	
				Ulcer excision + vagotomy	3			
				Underrunning	59			
				Ulcer excision	3	10[c]	26	
Kubba, 1996 [34]	Uncontrolled[b]	PU bleeding	36	Underrunning + vagotomy + pyloroplasty	24			
				Ulcer excision + vagotomy + pyloroplasty	3			
				Partial gastrectomy/antrectomy	9	3	14	Aggressive approach
				Underrunning	28	23	23	
				Ulcer excision	3			
Hunt, 1990 [35]	Uncontrolled[b]	DU bleeding	81	Partial gastrectomy, BII	81	10	12	
			101	Underrunning + vagotomy + pyloroplasty	101	17	10	Underrunning + vagotomy

Reference	Design	Indication	n	Procedure	n			Comment
Kuttila, 1991 [19]	Uncontrolled[b]	GU bleeding	58	Partial gastrectomy	58	3	2	Partial gastrectomy
			17	Ulcer excision + vagotomy	12	12	24	
		DU bleeding	42	Partial gastrectomy ± vagotomy	5	0	12	
			27	Partial gastrectomy ± vagotomy	42	19	22	
				Underruning + vagotomy + pyloroplasty	27			
Dousset, 1995 [36]	Uncontrolled[b]	PU bleeding	63	Oversewing/ulcer excision	29			
				Oversewing/ulcer excision + vagotomy	34	30	24	Radical approach
			15	Antrectomy + vagotomy	10	0	13	
					5			

Abbreviations: BI, Billroth I; BII, Billroth II; DU, duodenal ulcer; GU, gastric ulcer; PU, peptic ulcer.
[a] Analysis based on treatment received
[b] Subgroup analysis with analysis of comparability of study groups.
[c] Fatal rebleeding.
From Ohmann C, Imhof M, Röher H-D. Trends in peptic ulcer bleeding and surgical treatment. World J Surg 2000;24:284; with permission.

The operations

There are any number of procedures and operations that have been devised to treat ulcer disease and its complications. As was mentioned earlier, there is a fascinating history in the development of these operations. And, as with most matters of historical development in surgery, there is an unfortunate and unwieldy collection of eponyms associated with these procedures. Although the author personally finds that an understanding of how surgical problems were solved and by whom is a useful part of developing a working knowledge in our craft, I also believe that our discipline would benefit from confining our terminology to such as would minimize the likelihood of confusion. Perhaps we should take a lesson from airline pilots, as the Institute of Medicine, in their evaluation of medical error, has suggested. To that end, it might behoove us to establish some definitions before undertaking a discussion of possible operations.

Truncal vagotomy is the division of both of the vagus nerves above its first branches to the fundus of the stomach. The term vagectomy is sometimes used synonymously, albeit erroneously, with vagotomy. Vagectomy implies the resection of a piece of the vagus nerve, which is actually good practice when dividing the vagal trunk to confirm that the correct structure has been identified. Removing bits of nerve for pathologic evaluation during other kinds of vagus disrupting procedures is generally not done. Because the literature is replete with references to "truncal vagotomy," the author uses that term for the sake of discussion in this article. Unless otherwise specified, truncal vagotomy does imply division of both the posterior and anterior vagus nerves. When only one of the nerves is divided, it is usually the posterior branch. Posterior vagotomy is usually associated with another procedure, such as an anterior seromyotomy.

Selective vagotomy refers to complete division of the gastric branches of the vagus nerve—including the nerve branches to the pylorus. The branches of the vagus to the liver and gallbladder are preserved, as are the branches to the intestine. Because the nerve fibers innervating the pylorus (the nerves of Laterjet) are defeated, a concomitant gastric drainage procedure, gastroenterostomy or pyloroplasty, is also required. This operation has never been common in North America. Highly selective vagotomy (HSV) refers to division of the gastric branches of the vagus nerves that innervate the acid-producing portion of the stomach. When this operation is based upon anatomic landmarks, it is also referred to as a proximal gastric vagotomy (PGV). When HSV is performed on the basis of intraoperative pH evaluation, it is referred to as a parietal cell vagotomy (PCV). Methods of evaluating intraoperative gastric acid secretion include intragastric pH monitoring or instillation of intragastric Congo red dye.

Gastric resections and reconstructions suffer from the same degree of eponym usage, but our common parlance has been more likely to continue them in use. Gastric antrectomy refers to resection of the distal, gastrin-secreting, portion of the stomach. When primary reconstruction is performed by an end-to-end gastroduodenostomy, it is referred to as a Billroth I type procedure. When the duodenal stump is closed blindly, or over a drain, and the stomach is anastomosed to the jejunum in end-to-side gastrojejunostomy fashion, it is referred to as a Billroth II type reconstruction. Furthermore, if part of the width of the stomach is used in the anastomosis, it is referred to as Hofmeister type gastroenterostomy; whereas if the entire width of the stomach is used, it is referred to as a Polya type gastroenterostomy. Resection of the antrum can also be accompanied by gastroenterostomy to a defunctionalized limb of jejunum, referred to as a Roux-en-Y gastroenterostomy, named after the Swiss surgeon Cesar Roux. Although these eponyms give us all adequate opportunity to show what we have learned about these historical events, they may occasionally obscure the importance of why the different techniques matter. The eponyms associated with pyloroplasty are discussed later in this article.

Local procedures

Local excision of ulcers was first described by Czerny in 1882. Based on the early experience of high recurrence rates for local gastric ulcer and duodenal ulcer excisions, these lesser procedures were largely abandoned. In the modern era of pharmacologic control of acid secretion and eradication of *H pylori*, these procedure have not been re-evaluated. The main indication for limited resection of gastric ulcer is in the evaluation of the Type I and Type IV gastric ulcers to rule out malignancy.

Perforated ulcers may be managed by local measures. Although simple apposition of the ulcer has been described, this may be technically difficult to perform because of surrounding induration of tissue. The author does not recommend it. Omental patch has been described to "close" perforated ulcers. A simple omental patch can be created by fashioning, if necessary, a tongue of omentum and securing the tissue over the perforation with absorbable sutures. This technique, sometimes referred to as a "Graham patch" (Fig. 1) was actually first described by Cellen-Jones in 1929 [24]. Graham's description, reported in 1937 [25], involved suturing of a piece of omentum "either free or attached" without attempt at closing the perforation.

Management of ulcer hemorrhage by measures other than suturing, such as electrocautery, injection, and the like, are usually performed by endoscopic means. Ulcer hemorrhage significant enough to require operative management generally requires at least oversewing or under-running of the vessel with suture. The evidence addressing the need for concomitant acid-reducing procedure has been discussed previously in this article. The most important determinant of a successful procedure to control hemorrhage from ulcer is the ability to accurately locate the site or sites

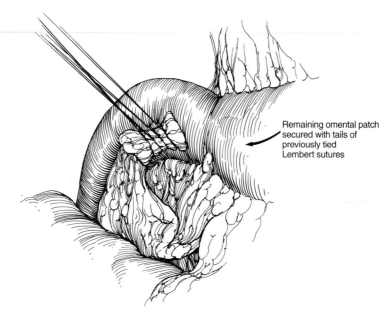

Fig. 1. Omental patch secured with Lembert sutures over duodenal perforation, referred to as Cellen-Jones procedure or Graham patch. (*From* Sabiston DC. Atlas of general surgery. Philadelphia: WB Saunders; 1994. p. 325; with permission.)

of hemorrhage. This is generally much easier to do endoscopically rather than by direct intra-operative inspection. The author very much tries to either perform or be present at endoscopy in "real time," to optimize understanding of the anatomic location of the source of hemorrhage. Bleeding associated with proximal duodenal ulcers is most commonly from penetrating posterior ulcers in the first portion of the duodenum that erode into the gastroduodenal artery. Under-running or oversewing of this vessel with nonabsorbable suture is described, as is suturing around the vessel in four quadrants. Care must be taken to not suture so deeply as to involve the distal common bile duct. Ligation of the gastroduodenal artery in continuity at the superior border of the pancreas may also be of benefit in controlling significant hemorrhage. Bleeding from gastric ulcers is usually manageable by excision of the bleeding ulcer.

Pyloroplasty

The pylorus is a circular layer of muscle that, in conjunction with the antrum, forms a mechanism that allows for the more effective mixing of gastric contents, and meters the rate of release of gastric contents into the duodenum. Its function is, to a large degree, mediated by the distal gastric branches of the vagus nerve known as the nerves of Laterjet. When the pylorus is scarred and fibrotic or the nerve supply to it is damaged, either a mechanical or functional gastric outlet obstruction will ensue. Pyloric obstruction can be mechanically addressed by resection of the pylorus, separate gastroenterostomy, or pyloroplasty.

Longitudinal incision of the pylorus with transverse closure was independently described by Heinecke and von Mikulicz in 1886 and 1887, respectively [26]. This technique is nearly always referred to as a Heinecke-Mikulicz pyloroplasty (Fig. 2). Jaboulay described a side-to-side gastro-duodenostomy (Fig. 3), which functionally bypasses the stenotic or obstructing pylorus, in 1892 [27]. This was later also described by von Mikulicz in 1898 [28]. The Jaboulay "pyloroplasty" was modified by Finney by incising through the pylorus and creating a single lumen in 1902 [28]. The performance of a Finney or Jaboulay type pyloroplasty is vanishingly rare in this era. Despite rare usage, these techniques frequently come up in conversation, particularly among professors and residents.

Pyloroplasty can also be performed by minimally invasive techniques. The standard Heinecke-Mikulicz type pyloroplasty can be performed with intracorporeal suturing techniques. Alternatively, one can create an anterior longitudinal gastrotomy through which an end-to-end-anstomosing (EEA) stapler device can be inserted. The pyloric ring can then be placed in the stapler, and a section of the pylorus can be excised and closed simultaneously, thereby breaking the ring. After the EEA device is removed, the gastrotomy can be closed by suture technique or linear staple closure.

Partial gastrectomy and restoration of foregut continuity

Resection of the gastric antrum will remove the gastrin-secreting cells of the stomach. Occasionally antral resection is necessary because of the presence of a significant prepyloric ulcer. Although Billroth first performed this operation of distal gastrectomy with gastroduodenostomy for a gastric cancer, its main indication is for a prepyloric ulcer with normal duodenum. Many modifications to this operation have been described by Rydiger, Kocher, Mayo, and others, but it is still generally referred to as a Billroth I procedure (Fig. 4). The proximal limit of gastric resection is based upon anatomic assessment, usually from the incisura along the lesser curve to a point on the greater curve of the stomach. The degree of adequate distal margin is to include normal duodenum just distal to the pylorus. Among the advantages of this operation is the preservation of "linear" foregut anatomy. With the availability of flexible fiber-optic endoscopy, this may be more important than in Billroth's day.

A problem associated with the Billroth I procedure is size mismatch between the gastric pouch and the duodenum. Partial closure of the stomach with associated gastroduodenostomy, using the remaining width of the divided edge of stomach, creates an intersection of suture lines known as the

A

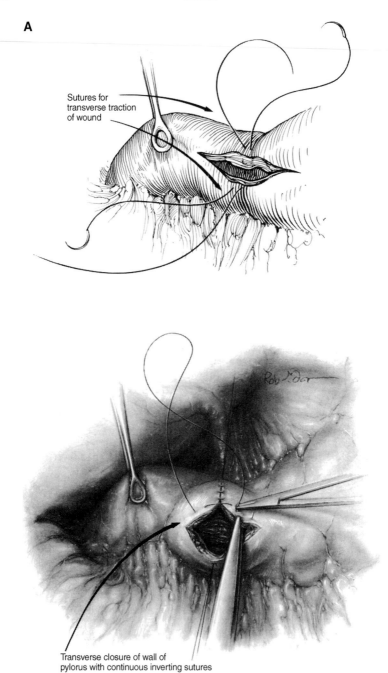

Sutures for
transverse traction
of wound

Transverse closure of wall of
pylorus with continuous inverting sutures

Fig. 2. Longitudinal incision through pylorus (*A*) followed by two-layer horizontal sutured closer (*B*), commonly referred to as a Heinecke-Mickulicz pyloroplasty. (*From* Sabiston DC. Atlas of general surgery. Philadelphia: WB Saunders; 1994. p. 252–3; with permission.)

B

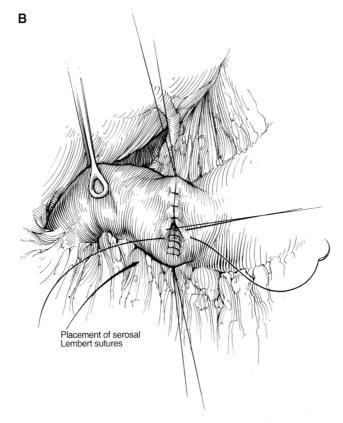

Placement of serosal
Lembert sutures

Fig. 2 (*continued*)

"angle of grief" or "jammerecke" [26]. Several alternative approaches to this problem have been offered, including "funneling" of the stomach with plicating sutures and then creating an end-to-end anastomosis.

Another problem that can be associated with the Billroth I operation is inadequate length for a tension-free reconstruction. This is most often the case with duodenal ulcers. For this reason, the Billroth II procedure gained usage. This procedure allows for a tension-free anastomosis to be created by anastomosing the divided stomach to the jejunum. The most common modifications of this procedure used are those described by Hofmeister in 1905 (a partial-width gastrojejunostomy) (Fig. 5) and Polya in 1911 (a full-width gastrojejunostomy) [26]. Although this operation eliminates, in theory, a tensioned anastomosis, it is still associated with some potential problems. Retained antrum creating a persistent hypergastrinemic state, afferent loop syndrome, and reflux of bile into the stomach—problems shared with the Billroth I procedure—are all possible, as are problems with the duodenal stump. The first problems are related to technical error. Because scarring can obscure the peripyloric anatomy, it is always

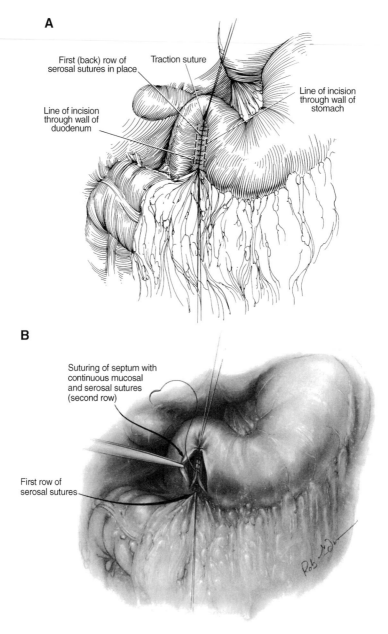

A

First (back) row of
serosal sutures in place

Traction suture

Line of incision
through wall of
stomach

Line of incision
through wall of
duodenum

B

Suturing of septum with
continuous mucosal
and serosal sutures
(second row)

First row of
serosal sutures

Fig. 3. (*A*) Closure of back wall of gastroduodenostomy and lines of proposed incision. (*B*) Running closure of inner layer of gastroduodenostomy and (*C*) closure of anterior external layer of pyloroplasty with Lembert sutures. (*From* Sabiston DC. Atlas of general surgery. Philadelphia: WB Saunders; 1994. p. 259–60; with permission.)

c

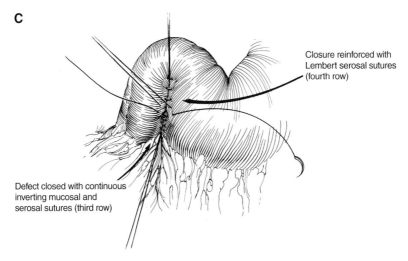

Closure reinforced with
Lembert serosal sutures
(fourth row)

Defect closed with continuous
inverting mucosal and
serosal sutures (third row)

Fig. 3 (*continued*)

imperative that the histological confirmation of duodenum be secured when performing an antrectomy with Billroth II type resection: retained gastric antrum will secrete gastrin in the absence of inhibitory feedback from the flow of acid. The problem of afferent loop syndrome may result from creating an overly long segment of jejunum proximal to the gastro-enterostomy. This may promote bacterial overgrowth or develop mechanical obstruction. This complication is best avoided by using the shortest length of jejunum between the ligament of Treitz and the anastomosis that is possible without tension.

Reflux of bile into the stomach is expected to some degree with both the Billroth I and Billroth II procedures. Bile gastritis can result, as can bile esophagitis if the gastric pouch is small or the lower esophageal sphincter is incompetent. There are two most commonly used strategies to avoid significant bile gastritis. The first is side-to-side jejunojejunostomy, described by Braun in 1892. The other is creation of an isoperistaltic defunctionalized jejunal limb with proximal gastric anastomosis to the distal limb of jejunum and proximal jejunum anastomosed to the distal limb of jejunum approximately 45 cm distal to the gastroenterostomy (Fig. 6)—known as a Roux-en-Y reconstruction [28]. The side-to-side Braun enteroenterostomy is performed between the afferent and efferent jejunal limbs to the gastrojejunal anastomosis. It is incompletely diverting of bile from the stomach, and in the author's experience, is associated with creating more problems than it solves. I would, however, concede that in cases of obstructing and unresectable processes of the intestines, such as are seen in some advanced malignancies or secondary to radiation injury, the Braun technique can be exceptionally useful.

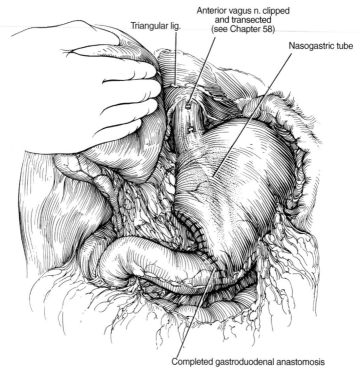

Anterior vagus n. clipped
and transected
(see Chapter 58)

Triangular lig.

Nasogastric tube

Completed gastroduodenal anastomosis

Fig. 4. Completed Billroth I gastroduodenostomy with partial closure of stomach and anterior vagectomy shown. (*From* Sabiston DC. Atlas of general surgery. Philadelphia: WB Saunders; 1994. p. 271; with permission.)

The problem of the duodenal stump is associated with both the Billroth II and Roux-en-Y type procedures. Numerous techniques for stump closure have been described. Independent of the suture material or technique of closure a few principles endure. Quality tissue must be used to secure a competent closure; a closure of potentially lesser quality tissue is probably best accompanied by the use of a duodenostomy tube and extraluminal drain; and if the antrum has been resected, the ulcer does not need to be excised. This last principle is credited to Finsterer as early as 1918 [28].

Operations for proximal, or high, gastric ulcers deserve separate comment. These ulcers are also referred to as Type IV gastric ulcers. Reports from the United States and Europe suggest that Type IV gastric ulcers represent less than 5% of all gastric ulcers [29]; however, the proximal gastric ulcer is reported in as high as 27% of patients who have gastric ulcer in Chile [9]. Numerous operations have been described to approach these high gastric ulcers, including local excision, partial gastrectomy with gastroduodenostomy or gastrojejunostomy, subtotal gastrectomy with esphagogastrojejunostomy, and mesogastrectomy with gastrogastrostomy. Also, a number of procedures directed toward improving gastric emptying

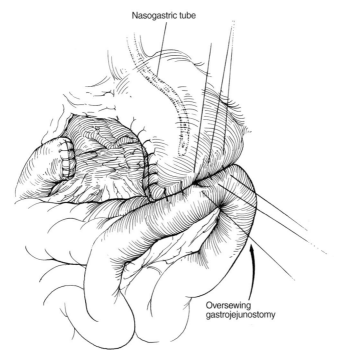

Nasogastric tube

Oversewing
gastrojejunostomy

Fig. 5. Antrectomy with Billroth II type gastrojejunostomy, Hofmeister technique, with oversewing of duodenal stump. (*From* Sabiston DC. Atlas of general surgery. Philadelphia: WB Saunders; 1994. p. 285; with permission.)

or acid suppression without excision of the ulcer have been described. In an excellent review by Csendes and colleagues [9], these operations are described in detail, as well as the short- and long-term results from these procedures.

Procedures to treat high gastric ulcer can be divided into two large groups: those that are associated with resection of the ulcer, and those that are not. The procedures that leave the ulcer in place are generally not recommended, because they are associated with complications such as recurrent hemorrhage. The procedures that involve resection of the ulcer are further categorized by a more precise description of the ulcer location. Ulcers located within 2 to 5 cm of the esophagogastric junction are considered subcardial, whereas those ulcers that are less than 2 cm away from the junction are called cardial or juxtaesophageal ulcers. For lesions that are juxtaesophageal, subtotal gastrectomy with esphagogastrojejunostomy (Csendes' procedure) is recommended. In this series [9], 23 patients were treated in this manner without mortality. For ulcers that were located between 2 and 5 cm from the esophagogastric junction, partial gastrectomy with gastrojejunostomy is recommended. It should be carefully stated that all of these procedures are considered for benign gastric ulcer, and do not

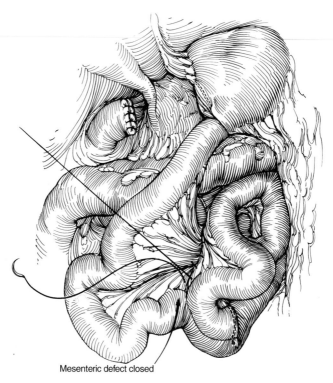

Mesenteric defect closed

Fig. 6. Antrectomy with Roux-en-Y gastrojejunostomy (ante-colic technique). (*From* Sabiston DC. Atlas of general surgery. Philadelphia: WB Saunders; 1994. p. 367; with permission.)

apply to ulcerated gastric malignancy. The discussion of the management of gastric cancer appears in the article by Dr. Munson elsewhere in this issue.

Vagal interruption

The glossary of terms used to describe vagal interruption procedures has been previously listed. For students of surgical history, a review of the experiments and experimenters who discovered these relationships makes for fascinating reading; however, a complete account of these adventures exceeds the scope of this article. The technical aspects of these operations are discussed further below.

Truncal vagotomy

Truncal vagotomy was introduced by Dragstedt and colleagues to attempt to eliminate the need for subtotal gastrectomy for effective treatment of ulcers [30]. The procedure requires division of the vagal trunks above the first branches to the gastric cardia and fundus, the criminal nerve of Grassi. The procedure may be performed through the left chest, the right chest, or the abdomen. Today it is most commonly approached through the abdomen, by either open or laparoscopic means. The phrenoesophageal ligament must be incised, allowing access to the distal esophagus. The left and right branches of the vagus, which run anteriorly and posteriorly, respectively, are then followed cephalad until the criminal nerves are identified. The author recommends performing an excision of a piece of each of the nerves (vagectomy) and sending each piece for histological confirmation. This will not ensure that the vagus has been divided in the right place, but if the pathological evaluation of the tissue is inconsistent with peripheral nerve, then it may be assumed that an incomplete vagotomy has been performed. Because truncal vagotomy will denervate the pylorus, a gastric drainage procedure should be simultaneously performed.

Highly selective vagotomy or proximal gastric vagotomy

HSV or PGV are vagal interrupting procedures that are designed to denervate the acid secreting portion of the stomach while leaving the vagal innervation to the pylorus intact, obviating the need for a gastric drainage procedure. A point on the stomach approximately 6 cm proximal to the pylorus is identified. Then the individual nerve fibers and concomitant blood vessels are serially divided along the lesser curve of the stomach, and followed for a distance of 5 to 6 cm along the esophagus, until all of the proximal vagal branches to the stomach are divided and the main vagal trunks remain intact. Pathological evaluation of nerve tissue plays no role here. This operation is also associated with a risk of devascularizing the lesser curve of the stomach. It also takes some time to do, depending upon the skill of the operative team. Incomplete division of the nerve fibers can adversely affect acid suppression, and excessive division can denervate the pylorus. To reduce the likelihood of incomplete vagotomy, some authors have advocated the use of intragastric pH measurement or testing with Congo red dye to assure adequate vagal disruption; this is then referred as PCV [31].

Selective vagotomy

Selective vagotomy (SV) is a rarely used operation that completely severs the gastric branches, including the pyloric branches, of the vagus nerves. This procedure leaves intact the vagal innervation to the liver and gallbladder, as well as the remainder of the intestinal innervation. The approach is similar to that used for PGV, with the addition of dividing the distal gastric branches. Pyloroplasty is performed routinely along with this procedure.

Posterior vagotomy and limited anterior vagal interruption

The use of minimally invasive techniques has reinvigorated the interest in operative management for acid suppression. Theoretically, an operation with limited trauma of access, limited need for intracorporeal reconstruction, and no requirement for bulky organ removal would be ideally suited for an alternative to chronic medical therapy. A laparoscopically achieved PGV would fit that description; however, the technical difficulty of that operation limits its utility. Posterior truncal vagotomy coupled with anterior seromyotomy may achieve a balance in efficacy and technical ease. Dissection for posterior vagotomy is performed in a similar fashion as described for truncal vagotomy. The posterior branch of the vagus is divided proximally to the criminal nerve. The anterior vagal branches to the gastric wall are then divided with electrocautery, by incising into the gastric wall musculature through the serosa and suturing the gastric wall after complete division, and checking the stomach for leak [32]. Other authors have suggested dividing the anterior gastric wall with sequential linear stapling devices to disrupt the vagal branches and seal the gastric wall simultaneously [33]. Because the pylorus is innervated predominantly by the posterior branch of the vagus in a small percentage of patients, a pyloroplasty may be required. Some authors recommend performing a pyloroplasty in conjunction with this procedure routinely [30].

Outcomes

The literature has variably reported on the success of outcomes using the procedures previously described. There are many factors that may explain the variability of the reported results in the literature: when the report was written, failure to control for other contributing factors to success or failure, bias that may have been present in the opinions of the authors, and the cultural mood at the time of report. It would be nice to insert a table of definitive results here that one could turn to that lists the percentage of responders in one way or another; but the author thinks that may be an irresponsible act given the factors mentioned above. There are, however, some trends that I think we can allow to guide us in our decision-making.

One consistent trend is that complicated ulcers are less likely to recur if one eliminates the causative agent as well as manages the complication. Cessation of NSAID use and suppression of acid secretion are both associated with a decreased likelihood of ulcer recurrence. Eradication of *H pylori* appears to be associated with markedly reduced recurrence of bleeding or recurrence, as previously described. Operative suppression of acid secretion is associated with decreased persistence or recurrence of hemorrhage. Historically, the data suggested that a more aggressive suppression of acid secretion (ie, subtotal gastric resection) was more likely to prevent recurrence of hemorrhage than a lesser procedure such as limited antrectomy [8], and that eradication of neural stimulation of acid secretion allows for better results with lesser degrees of gastric resection [30]. Similarly, reduction of the degree of vagal interruption to the stomach is associated with an increase in the likelihood of ulcer recurrence or recurrence of hemorrhage. The other complications of more "radical" procedures, however (dumping, weight loss, anemia, diarrhea, bile gastritis, or gastric dysmotility) are all increased with a greater degree of gastric resection or vagal disruption—a classic series of trades. Whether these comparisons are all true in the modern era of pharmacologic proton pump inhibition and *H pylori* eradication remains to be seen.

Summary

The surgical management of patients who have acid peptic ulcers requires not only a firm understanding of the technical options, but an even firmer grasp of the anatomic, physiologic, and pathophysiologic relationships of the organs involved. If ever there were a constellation of problems in which the surgeon needs to be far more than a technician, this is it. The wealth of information that has been discovered on this subject, from the clinical observations of William Beaumont to the discovery of complex cellular biology and hormonal signaling, is enough to occupy the study of several careers. Although patients who have acid peptic disorders have largely become the primary responsibility of physicians and specialists other than surgeons, when significant complications occur in these patients, and they do, it is still the surgeon who is called upon to intervene.

References

[1] Sebastian M, Prem Chandran VP, El Ashaal YIM, et al. *Helicobacter pylori* infection in perforated peptic ulcer disease. Br J Surg 1995;82:360.
[2] Ohmann C, Imhof M, Röher H-D. Trends in peptic ulcer bleeding and surgical treatment. World J Surg 2000;24:284.
[3] Lee WJ, Wu MS, Chen Yuan RH, et al. Seroprevalence of *Helicobacter pylori* in patients with surgical peptic ulcer. Arch Surg 1997;132:430.
[4] Liu TJ, Wu CC. Peptic ulcer surgery: experience in Taiwan from 1982–1993. Asian J Surg 1997;20:305.
[5] Bliss DW, Stabile BE. The impact of ulcerogenic drugs on surgery for the treatment of peptic ulcer disease. Arch Surg 1991;126:609.
[6] Sonnenberg A. Peptic ulcer. In: Everhart JE, editor. Digestive diseases in the United States: epidemiology and impact. Washington (DC): US Department of Health and Human Services, National Institutes of Health publication no. 94–1447; 1994. p. 359.
[7] In: Everhart JH, editor. Digestive diseases in the United States: epidemiology and impact. National Digestive Diseases Data Working Group. Washington (DC): US Department of Health and Human Services, National Institutes of Health publication no. 94–1447; 1994. p. 457.
[8] Johnston D. Duodenal and gastric llcer. In: Schwartz SI, Elllis H, editors. Maingot's abdominal operations. 9th edition. Norwalk (CT): Appleton-Lange; 1989. p. 599.

[9] Csendes A, Braghetto I, Calvo F, et al. Surgical treatment of high gastric ulcer. Am J Surg 1985;149(6):765–70.

[10] Svanes C. Trends in perforated peptic ulcer: incidence, etiology, treatment and prognosis. World J Surg 2000;24:277.

[11] Svanes C, Lie RT, Kvåle G, et al. Incidence of perforated ulcer in western Norway 1935–1990: cohort or period dependent time trends? Am J Epidemiol 1995;141:836.

[12] Ng EKW, Chung SCS, Sung JJY, et al. High prevalence of *Helicobacter pylori* infection in duodenal ulcer perforations not caused by non-steroidal anti-inflammatory drugs. Br J Surg 1996;83:1779.

[13] Reinbach DH, Cruickshank G, McColl KEL. Acute perforated duodenal ulcer is not associated with *Helicobacter pylori* infections. Gut 1993;34:1344.

[14] Devereaux CE, Binmoeller KF. Endoclip: closing the surgical gap. Gastrointest Endosc 1999;50(3):440.

[15] Therapeutic endoscopy and bleeding ulcers: NIH consensus conference. JAMA 1989;262: 1369.

[16] Sugawa C, Steffes CP, Nakamura R, et al. Upper GI bleeding in an urban hospital: etiology, recurrence and prognosis. Ann Surg 1990;212:521.

[17] Poxon VA, Keighley MRB, Dykes PW, et al. Comparison of minimal and conventional surgery in patients with bleeding peptic ulcer: a multicentre trial. Br J Surg 1991;78:1344.

[18] Inadomi J, Koch J, Cello JP. Long-term follow-up of endoscopic treatment for bleeding gastric and duodenal ulcers. Am J Gastroenterol 1995;90:861.

[19] Kuttila K, Havia T, Pekkala E, et al. Surgery of acute peptic ulcer hemorrhage. Ann Chir Gynaecol 1991;80:26.

[20] Millat B, Hay JM, Valleur P, et al. French Associations for Surgical Research: emergency surgical treatment for bleeding duodenal ulcer: oversewing plus vagotomy versus gastric resection, a controlled randomized trial. World J Surg 1993;17:568.

[21] Jaspersen D, Koener T, Schorr W, et al. *Helicobacter pylori* eradication reduces the rate of rebleeding in ulcer hemorrhage. Gastrointest Endosc 1995;41:5.

[22] Rokkas T, Karameris A, Mavrogeorgis A, et al. Eradication of *Helicobacter pylori* reduces the possibility of rebleeding in peptic ulcer disease. Gastrointest Endosc 1995;41:1.

[23] Santander C, Gravalos RG, Cedenilla AG, et al. Maintenance treatment vs *Helicobacter pylori* eradication in preventing rebleeding of the peptic ulcer disease: a clinical trial and follow-up of two years [abstract]. Gastroenterolgy 1995;108:A208.

[24] Cellen-Jones CJ. A rapid method of treatment in perforated duodenal ulcer. BMJ 1929;1: 1076.

[25] Graham RR. The treatment of perforated duodenal ulcers. Surg Gynecol Obstet 1937;64: 235.

[26] Weil PH, Buchberger R. From Billroth to PCV: a century of gastric surgery. World J Surg 1999;23:736.

[27] Harkins HN, Nyhus LM. Surgery of the stomach and duodenum. 2nd edition. Boston: Little, Brown; 1969.

[28] Buchberger R, Kunz H. Zur Geschicte der Chirurgischen Behandlung des Magen-Zwoelffingerdam-Geschwers. Bruns Beitr Klin Chir 1968;216:2–4 [in German].

[29] Braasch JW, Cain JL, Priestley T. Juxtaesophageal gastric ulcer. Surg Gynecol Obstet 1955; 101:280.

[30] Donahue PE. Parietal cell vagotomy versus vagotomy-antrectomy: ulcer surgery in the modern era. World J Surg 2000;24:264.

[31] Donahue PE, Bombeck CT, Nyhus LM. The endoscopic Congo red test during proximal gastric vagotomy. Am J Surg 1987;153:249.

[32] Dubois F. New surgical strategy for gastroduodenal ulcer: Laparoscopic approach. World J Surg 2000;24:270.

[33] Gomez-Ferrer F. Gastrectomielineaire anterieure et vagotomy tronculaire posterieure par laparoscopie. Journal of Abdominal Surgery 1992;4:35 [in French].

[34] Kubba AK, Choudari C, Rajgopal C, et al. The outcome of surgery for major peptic ulcer haemorrhage following failed endoscopic therapy. Eur J Gastroenterol Hepatol 1996;8: 1175.

[35] Hunt PS, McIntyre RLE. Choice of emergency operative procedure for bleeding duodenal ulcer. Br J Surg 1990;77:1004.

[36] Dousset B, Suc B, Boudet MJ, et al. Surgical treatment of severe ulcerous hemorrhages: predictive factors of operative mortality. Gastroenterol Clin Biol 1995;19:259.

ELSEVIER
SAUNDERS

SURGICAL
CLINICS OF
NORTH AMERICA

Surg Clin N Am 85 (2005) 931–947

Current Status of Antireflux Surgery

Derick J. Christian, MD, Jo Buyske, MD*

*Department of Surgery, University of Pennsylvania Health System,
Penn Presbyterian Medical Center, 38th and Market Street Philadelphia, PA 19104, USA*

Surgery for gastroesophageal reflux disease (GERD) has been in a state of evolution over the last 70 years. Nissen's fundoplication, Belsey's wrap, and Hill's gastropexy have all been introduced, studied, and modified. Different approaches have been used, including thoracotomy, laparotomy, thoracoscopy, laparoscopy, and robotic-assisted techniques. The merits of medical versus surgical management of the disorder, the role of laparoscopy in first-time and redo surgery, the need for esophageal lengthening procedures and partial fundoplications, and more recently, the role of endoluminal therapies for GERD have all been debated extensively. We are surely still in the midst of this evolution. This article attempts to summarize where we have been, where we are, and where we might be going in the surgical management of GERD.

Historical aspects

Nissen

In 1936, Rudolph Nissen excised the cardia of the stomach in a patient who had an esophageal ulcer, and anastomosed the esophagus to the stomach. He buttressed the suture line by wrapping the fundus of the stomach around it and the lower esophagus. Years later Nissen astutely noted that the patient had no heartburn, and rightfully attributed that to the "wrap" used at his surgery. In 1955, Nissen applied his theory in the operating room and wrapped a patient who had reflux esophagitis [1]. In 1956 he reported his work in the Swiss journal, *Schweizerische Medizinische Wochenschrift* (Fig. 1) [2].

Allison

Before Nissens' work, hiatal hernia was thought to be the main cause of reflux [3]. It followed logically that reduction of hiatal hernia would restore

---

* Corresponding author.
E-mail address: Jo.buyske@uphs.upenn.edu (J. Buyske).

doi:10.1016/j.suc.2005.05.007
surgical.theclinics.com

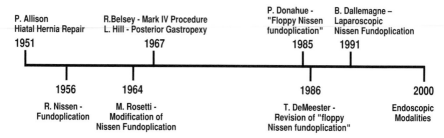

Fig. 1. Evolution of antireflux surgery.

the normal control mechanism, thus decreasing heartburn, reflux, and esophagitis. In 1951 Philip Allison [4] reported a technique for repair of hiatal hernia in the treatment of GERD. He described left thoracotomy, restoration of the abdominal length of the esophagus, posterior crural repair, and left phrenic nerve crush. The last was done to paralyze the left hemidiaphragm, causing eventration and securing the position of gastro-esophageal (GE) junction in the abdomen. The long-term results of this operation, however, were unsatisfactory. Allison reported a 20-year retro-spective survey of 553 patients operated on for various types of hiatal hernia [5]. Only 66% of the patients had symptomatic relief, and 49% had re-currence of the hiatal hernia.

Belsey

In Bristol, England, Ronald Belsey was also working on the problem of GE reflux. His initial operation underwent multiple modifications before the final version, Mark IV, in 1967 [6]. He called his technique the Mark IV as a reminder of the trial and error that had proceeded this final version. His repair emphasized physiology over anatomy. It was designed to restore all the normal functions of a competent cardia. Performed via a thoracotomy, his procedure emphasized mobilization of the esophagus and the cardia. The fundus was drawn through the chest to perform the 240° wrap, and then reduced back into the abdomen. Finally the crura were reapproximated to prevent a hiatal hernia. He theorized that the restoration of a 4- to 5-cm segment of the lower esophagus to the higher-pressure abdominal zone was essential in prevention of reflux.

Hill

Another important contributor was Lucius Hill. He demonstrated that the antireflux barrier consisted of the gastroesophageal valve, the lower esophageal sphincter (LES), the diaphragm, and posterior fixation of the gastroesophageal junction [7]. He initially demonstrated this in cadaver experiments. Later he used a retroflexed endoscope in live patients to demonstrate the mucoso-mucosal fold created by the entry of the esophagus into the stomach. His technique aimed to re-establish that 180° fold that was lost in patients who have severe reflux. Using an upper midline incision, he placed sutures between the proximal lesser curvature of the stomach, the median arcuate ligament, and the anterior and posterior phrenoesophageal fascial bundles. He included placement of cardio-diaphragmatic sutures for fixation of the GE junction, along with closure of the hiatus.

Nissen modifications

Nissen's original fundoplication included mobilization of the lower 5 to 8 cm of esophagus, and takedown of the gastrohepatic omentum, including the hepatic branch of the vagus nerve. The anterior and posterior walls of the fundus were wrapped around the esophagus (Fig. 2). Since that initial description, multiple modifications have been made. For example, Nissen and Rossetti suggested tightening the wrap in very obese patients by using only the anterior fundic wall [8].

A large experience with Nissen fundoplication was gained (Table 1) [9–14]). Polk and Zeppa [9] reported a series of 994 patients, 96% of whom reported symptomatic improvement during a short follow-up period of

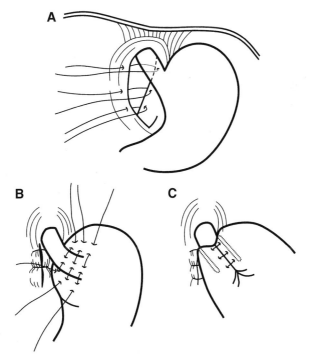

Fig. 2. Performing Nissen fundoplication. (*A*) Sutures to reapproximate the crura. (*B*) Sutures taken in the anterior wall of the fundus to perform the wrap. (*C*) Completed Nissen fundoplication.

Table 1
Large series of Nissen fundoplication

Study	Year	No. of patients	Length of follow-up (years)	% patients symptoms free
Polk and Zeppa [9]	1971	994	2.5	96.0
Rossetti and Heill [10]	1977	590	Not available	87.5
Bushkin et al [11]	1976	165	10	92.0
Nicholson and Nohl-Oser [12]	1976	141	12	97.1
Negre et al [13]	1983	94	10	81.0
Ellis and Crozier [14]	1984	82	5.75	90.0

2.5 years. Rossetti and Heill [10] reported their series of 590 patients. They showed improvement of symptoms in 87.5% of the patients. These reports confirmed efficacy, but also reported significant postoperative problems. Dysphagia and gas bloat syndrome were issues of major concern. Woodward and colleagues [15] noted postoperative dysphagia in 24% of the patients. Furthermore, gas bloat syndrome was reported in 54% of the patients. This decreased to 21% after 1 year, and 11% after a longer follow-up period.

In an effort to address these issues, Philip Donahue introduced the "floppy Nissen fundoplication" in a dog model [16]. Using a 15 Hegar dilator underneath the fundoplication and a 50 French esophageal bougie during the creation of the fundoplication, he ensured a standard, large diameter to the wrap. In 1985 he reported 8-year follow-up of 77 patients who had floppy Nissen fundoplication [17]. Ninety-seven percent of patients were symptom-free. Only 2 patients reported the adverse effect of gas bloat syndrome and inability to belch.

Dr. Tom DeMeester further modified this technique in his landmark study in 1986 [18]. He used a 60 French esophageal bougie, shortened the fundoplication length to 1 cm, and performed complete mobilization of the gastric fundus with division of the short gastric vessels. His group reported that 91% of patients remained symptom-free in a 10-year follow-period. Importantly, the incidence of persistent dysphagia was decreased from 21% to 3%.

In the 1960s, Gurner [19], Menguy [20], and Toupet [21] all worked on modifications that allowed the partial fundoplication of Belsey's Mark IV to be done through the abdomen instead of the more morbid thoracic approach (Fig. 3). These approaches had in common mobilization of the abdominal portion of the esophagus, narrowing of the crura, and finally a partial fundoplication, suturing the gastric fundus to the esophagus.

Partial versus total fundoplication

Advocates of partial fundoplication claim that it results in fewer side effects than a 360° fundoplication. Complications such as gas bloat and

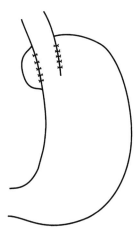

Fig. 3. Schematic of posterior partial fundoplication.

persistent dysphagia appear to be less frequent. Partial fundoplication was recommended as the initial procedure of choice for patients who have poor esophageal motility [22]. Patients suffering from postoperative dysphagia had their 360° wraps revised to partial fundoplication [23]. Some authors propose partial wraps as the operation of choice, regardless of esophageal motility [24].

Unfortunately, long-term follow-up revealed a high failure rate of partial wraps in terms of control of acid reflux. Jobe and coworkers [25] showed a worse outcome with a partial fundoplication than with total fundoplication. Other authors noted that as many as 50% of the patients who had partial fundoplication had evidence of reflux when studied postoperatively [26].

Minimally invasive era

Bernard Dallemagne and coworkers [27] reported the first laparoscopic Nissen fundoplication in 1991. Cushieri and colleagues [28] subsequently reported a multicenter trial of 116 patients undergoing laparoscopic fundoplication. Randomized trials showed there to be a benefit to the laparoscopic approach [29]. John Hunter at Emory University in Atlanta, Georgia and Jeff Peters at the University of Southern California in Los Angeles, among others, developed standardized approaches and pro-spectively gathered data bases to follow the outcomes. Since then, many single-center trials have been published (Table 2) [30–35].

Initial nonrandomized studies comparing open and laparoscopic approaches to fundoplication suggested that although the laparoscopic approach took more time to perform, the incidence of postoperative complications such as incisional pain and respiratory compromise was

Table 2
Single center laparoscopic Nissen fundoplication trials

Study	Year	Number of patients	OR time (minutes)	F/U period (months)	% patients symptom free
Hinder et al [30]	1994	198	150	32	97.0
Jamieson et al [31]	1994	155	120	3	97.1
Hunter et al [32]	1996	252	185	17	93.0
Gotley et al [33]	1996	200	149	12	99.5
Watson et al [34]	1996	174	80	3	91.0
Cattey et al [35]	1996	100	101	19	90.0

Abbreviations: F/U, follow-up; OR, operating room.

lower, and postoperative disability and hospital stay were shorter. Since then, multiple randomized studies also have been performed (Table 3) [36–40]. In 1997, Laine and coworkers [40] reported a randomized trial of 110 patients comparing laparoscopic versus open Nissen fundoplication. Esophageal monitoring and pH recording were performed during both the preoperative and postoperative periods. During the 3-month follow-up period, 24-hour pH tracing was normal in 97% of the patients in the laparoscopic Nissen fundoplication group and 68% of the patients in the open group. Likewise, LES pressure had increased by 80% in the laparoscopic group and only 40% in the open group. The mean duration of the operation was 88 minutes in the laparoscopic group and 57 minutes in the open group. The average hospital stay was 3.2 days in the laparoscopic

Table 3
Randomized trials of open vs. laparoscopic Nissen fundoplication

Study	Year	F/U period	Number patients	OR time (min)	(%) Postop pain	Postop hospital stay (days)	(%) patients with severe heartburn
Nilson et al [36]	2004	5 years	17 lap	na	na	na	6
			23 open				4
Ackreyd et al [37]	2004	12 months	52 lap	82	4	3	8
			47 open	46	30	5	2
Chrysos et al [38]	2002	3 months	56 lap	77	5	2	4
			50 open	83	92	6	2
Wenner et al [39]	2001	6 months	30 lap	na	na	na	4
			30 open				7
Laine et al [40]	1997	3 months	55 lap	88	na	3	0
			55 open	57		6	4

Abbreviations: lap, laparoscopic; na, not available; postop, postoperative.

group, versus an average 6.4-day stay in the open group. Similarly in 2002, Chrysos and colleagues [38] reported a randomized trial of laparoscopic versus open Nissen fundoplication in 106 patients. This showed the open group to have more pain as well as more frequent respiratory complications. At 12-month follow-up, both open and laparoscopic groups were shown to have increased lower LES tone. Follow-up pH monitoring confirmed reduction of reflux in both groups as well.

Patient selection

In the properly selected patient, laparoscopic antireflux surgery with a short, floppy fundoplication has a success rate of greater than 90% in addressing the classic symptoms of reflux, specifically heartburn and regurgitation [41]. Patients who have atypical presenting symptoms such as cough, hoarseness, or mouth burning are less likely to have relief of these complaints [42]. The patient most likely to do well has been fairly clearly delineated, and can be identified with a thorough evaluation.

A good history elicits all reflux-related symptoms, as well as all symptoms the patient may wrongly attribute to reflux. The authors routinely ask extensive questions about the nature, timing, and duration of heartburn symptoms. We ask about temporal relationships to eating, lying down, bending over, or stress. We discuss habits of air swallowing, gum chewing, caffeine ingestion, and cigarette smoking. We also ask about lower digestive symptoms such as abdominal pain, constipation, diarrhea, or flatulence. Extraesophageal symptoms such as cough, especially night cough, throat clearing, sinus infections, pneumonias, dental caries, and pneumonias should be sought.

A history of abdominal pain bears more discussion and evaluation. The authors have a low threshold for getting a sonogram of the right upper quadrant to look for gallstones as a potential cause of this, and a low threshold as well for cholecystectomy at the time of antireflux surgery should gallstones be present. Constipation and diarrhea should elicit a search for either inflammatory bowel disease, if appropriate, or irritable bowel syndrome, which may be a poor prognostic indicator for results from reflux surgery [43,44].

Complaints of bloating, postprandial distention, and dyspepsia should raise the suspicion of delayed gastric emptying as a contributing factor in reflux [45,46]. A gastric emptying study should be obtained to confirm or refute the existence of this disorder. If present, these patients should be counseled about the risk of gas bloat symptoms after fundoplication. In mild to moderate cases, fundoplication may actually increase the rate of gastric emptying [47]. In severe cases, consideration should be given to adding a gastric emptying procedure to the operation.

Upper airway symptoms need to be addressed carefully. To date we have a very poor ability to predict which patients who have a primary extraesophageal complaint will respond well to antireflux surgery [48,49]. An exhaustive search for other causes should be undertaken, and objective proof of the simultaneous presence of reflux is mandatory. Good symptom correlation to episodes of reflux on a 24-hour pH study may be reassuring, but we still have no sure way of separating responders from nonresponders. The patient must clearly understand this, and be a partner in the decision-making should a decision be made to proceed.

Response to medication has been shown to be a valuable prognostic indicator [50]. This can be assessed qualitatively by simply asking patients if their medications make them feel better, and if they feel worse when they are stopped. Acid suppression is often withheld for several days before 24 hour pH testing, which can provide a useful window for this assessment.

Diagnostic studies

The core group of studies consists of upper gastrointestinal endoscopy (EGD), upper gastrointestinal fluoroscopy with barium, 24-hour pH testing, and esophageal manometry.

EGD allows examination of the esophageal mucosa. It is useful in identifying the presence of esophagitis and grading the severity. Endoscopy can help identify other pathology, such as diverticula, hiatal hernia, webs, rings, or strictures. Tissue biopsies to screen for Barrett's esophagus and esophagitis should be obtained. EGD is less useful in stratifying the size or significance of a hiatal hernia, and should not be exclusively relied upon for that information.

The 24-hour pH test is the gold standard for presence of pathologic reflux. A small catheter bearing a pH probe at its end is placed transnasally. The tip is positioned 5 cm above the LES, with additional probes placed in the stomach and 15 cm above the LES. Quantitative measures of esophageal acid exposure are made every 4 to 6 seconds. The patient activates an event marker in response to symptoms, meals, and body position changes. The catheter remains in place for 24 hours. Multiple parameters can be calculated. These include total number of reflux episodes, duration of the longest reflux episode, and percentage of total time the esophageal pH is less than 4 [51]. The "DeMeester score" is obtained by combining these results. Normal individuals have a DeMeester score of 14 or less [52]. It is important to note that this is a relative scale, and there is no absolute value that clearly identifies pathologic GERD.

Use of the 24-hour pH probe is somewhat limited by the patient's ability to tolerate a small catheter down the nose for 24 hours. An alternative is a probe that is attached endoscopically to the mucosa 6 cm above the GE junction. It gathers pH data for 2 days. During the next 10 to 14 days it detaches itself form the mucosa. Because there is only a single probe, it provides less information than the traditional 24-hour pH probe; however, it may be better tolerated in some patients.

Esophageal manometry should also be routinely performed. It provides information on the function of the LES and esophageal body. The ideal candidate for surgery has a mechanically defective sphincter. Stein, DeMeester, and Naspetti [53] looked at the LES of 50 normal individuals and also of 622 patients who had GERD. They arrived at the following criteria for a defective LES: mean pressure less than 6 mm/Hg, overall length less than 2 cm. and intra-abdominal length less than 1 cm. Esophageal manometry may also identify patients who have abnormal esophageal motility, such as achalasia or scleroderma. Other patients who have ineffective or absent peristalsis may be candidates for a partial fundoplication, or may be better served avoiding operation all together.

Barium esophagram is the most useful test to delineate the anatomy of esophagus. It aids in identifying the length of the esophagus and the presence or absence of a hiatal hernia, both of which will influence the procedure of choice. Barium esophagram can also identify subtle stricture or Shatski's rings, which may not be apparent on endoscopy.

Short esophagus

The entity of short esophagus warrants some discussion. There is no consensus in the literature on the incidence, definition, or even the very existence of short esophagus. In theory, severe and chronic exposure to acid produces fibrosis and esophageal shortening. This may compromise the ability of the surgeon to reduce the GE junction into the abdomen, or to keep it there for the long term. Historically the incidence of short esophagus has been variously reported as ranging from 60%, as described by Pearson and Todd [54], to 0% as reported by Hill and coworkers [55]. More recently, two large studies reported the incidence of short esophagus requiring an esophageal lengthening procedure to be 3% to 4%[56,57].

Several authors have attempted to identify factors that would allow the diagnosis of short esophagus before surgery. Awad and colleagues [58] looked at variables such as endoscopic evidence of stricture, Barrett's esophagus, irreducible hernia greater than 5 cm, and esophageal shortening on manometric studies. The group concluded that only endoscopic evidence of stricture or Barrett's esophagus was associated with a short esophagus. Gastel and coworkers [59] also concluded that only esophageal stricture predicted short esophagus. At this time, the only reliable way to exclude a short esophagus is at surgery. An effective antireflux valve requires 2.5 to 3 cm of intra-abdominal esophagus [60]. If the distal esophagus cannot be brought fairly easily below the diaphragm, then there is a presumptive diagnosis of short esophagus.

Multiple operations have been described for the management of the shortened esophagus. These include intrathoracic fundoplication, esophageal lengthening procedures, or ultimately, esophagectomy. Collis initially described an esophageal lengthening procedure using a thoracoabdominal incision for esophageal mobilization. He established additional length by dividing the proximal stomach in line with the esophagus, a Collis gastroplasty [60]. Pearson and Henderson [61] later described a transthoracic Collis gastroplasty combined with Belsey's fundoplication. A series of 26 patients showed that 76% were symptom free at 5- to 12-year follow-up. Orringer combined the Collis gastroplasty with a Nissen fundoplication, a transthoracic Collis-Nissen procedure. He demonstrated reflux control in 88% of 261 patients during a 10-year follow-up period [62]. Steichen [63] later introduced the use of circular and linear staplers to create an abdominal Collis-Nissen procedure. In 1996, Swanstrom and colleagues [56] described a combined laparoscopic/thoracoscopic Collis gastroplasty, which, though effective, was not widely adopted. Johnson and coworkers [57] described a totally laparoscopic Collis gastroplasty using staplers in 1998. A short follow-up period of 6 weeks showed symptomatic improvement in 93% of the 15 patients.

Mesh repair of hiatal hernia

Some authors have looked at the use of prosthetic material for the reapproximation of the hiatus. This would create an intense scar that might prevent wrap migration or disruption of the crural repair. The proponents of this method report a significant decrease in hernia recurrence. Frantzides and colleagues [64] showed a significant decrease in recurrence rate by using prosthetic material for hiatal defects greater then 8 cm. Champion's group [65] showed the same results in patients who had hernias of 5 cm. The same group proposes the use of prosthetic material routinely for redo-fundoplication. Granderath and coworkers [66] reported the use of poly-propylene mesh in 24 patients undergoing laparoscopic redo-fundoplication. Concern about the potential for complication related to mesh in this position has limited adoption of this approach. There is no consensus in the surgical community on this subject.

Technique

The patient is placed in a supine split-leg position. This allows the surgeon to stand in the midline between the patient's legs. Access to the abdominal cavity is obtained with either a Veress needle or a Hassan technique. A standard five-port technique is used (Fig. 4). The authors begin the dissection by opening the bare area of the gastrohepatic ligament, taking care to preserve the hepatic branch of the vagus nerve whenever possible. The phrenoesophageal ligament is lifted off the esophagus and divided. The retroesophageal space is then opened by sweeping down the right side of the hiatus until the left leaflet of the crus is seen behind the esophagus. The left leaflet is then likewise swept clean, effectively encircling the esophagus without actually dissecting near it. With aid of an atraumatic esophageal

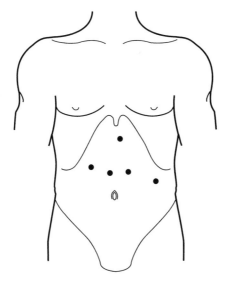

Fig. 4. Port placement sites for laparoscopic antireflux surgery.

retractor or soft rubber drain, the esophagus is freed of its mediastinal attachments to obtain at least 4 cm of intra-abdominal length. The short gastric vessels are then taken down completely with the aid of a harmonic scalpel. A short, loose fundoplication is created over a 60 French bougie. A nasogastric tube is left in position.

The patient is kept in-house overnight. Antiemetic medications are given liberally. The nasogastric tube is removed the next day. The patient is started on clear liquids and advanced rapidly to a soft-solid diet. The patient is discharged when tolerating a diet, usually on postoperative day 1 or 2. The authors do not obtain any routine postoperative testing in house. The first postoperative visit is 2 weeks after surgery, at which point the diet can be liberalized if there is no dysphagia. A second visit is scheduled 6 weeks after surgery. An esophagram is obtained at 1 year, and repeated annually for 5 years, with annual office visits as well. Twenty-four hour pH studies should be done if there is any question of recurrent or persistent reflux.

Surgical failure

Failed surgery is heralded by recurrence or persistence of preoperative symptoms, or occurrence of new symptoms after an antireflux operation. The most common symptom is dysphagia [67]. Other commonly reported symptoms are early satiety, abdominal bloating, diarrhea, and recurrent reflux symptoms. Subjective reporting of symptoms, however, has very poor correlation with postoperative acid reflux. In one study [68], the positive predictive value of heartburn after reflux surgery was only 43%, although a negative predictive value was 82%. A careful and thorough evaluation must be performed in a patient who has postoperative symptoms.

The first test to undertake when a patient complains of symptoms postoperatively is a video barium esophagram. In good hands this provides both anatomic and functional information. Radiologic abnormalities after antireflux procedures have been categorized into Types I, II, III, and IV failures (Fig. 5) [69]. Type I is a complete disruption of the fundoplication, with recurrence of the hiatal hernia. Type II is part of the stomach slipped above the diaphragm. Type III represents part of the stomach above the fundoplication but below the diaphragm. Finally, Type IV is the herniation of the fundoplication through the hiatus into the chest.

Beyond wrap disruption or displacement, other reasons for failure of antireflux surgery include breakdown of crural closure or inadequate closure at surgery, and perhaps lack of adequate mobilization of the esophagus. Some investigators report that failure to divide the short gastric vessels may be a cause of failure [70].

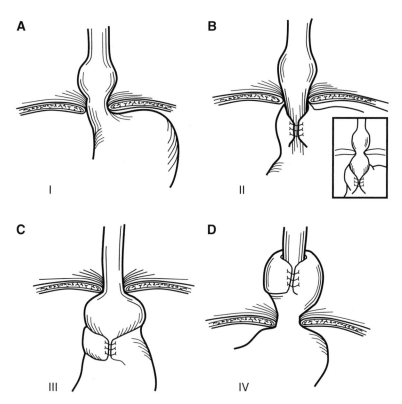

Fig. 5. (A–D) Anatomic failures of fundoplication. (Modified from Hinder RA: Gastroesoph-ageal reflux disease. In: Bell RH Jr, Rikkers LF, Mulholland MW, editors. Digestive tract surgery: a text and atlas. Philadelphia: Lippincott-Raven Publishers; 1996. p. 19; with permission.)

Body habitus has also been implicated in the failure of fundoplication. Perez and colleagues [71] recently evaluated 224 patients after laparoscopic Nissen and open Belsey Mark IV repair. Patients who had a body mass index of greater than 30 had a significantly higher symptomatic recurrence rate (27%) then those who had a body mass index of less than 29 (8%).

Redo surgery

Persistent or new troublesome symptoms after an antireflux procedure warrant a careful evaluation. Investigation should be directed at both the original preoperative evaluation and the current situation. The initial evalution should be reviewed with an eye toward any predisposing problems. Esophageal manometry might show borderline function predisposing to persistent symptoms postoperatively. Review of the original 24-hour pH test might show poor symptom correlation, which suggests that postoperative symptoms may be due to something other than recurrent reflux. The operative report should be obtained and reviewed, with attention to such details as esophageal length, use of a bougie or dilator to size the wrap, closure of the hiatus, and division of the short gastric vessels. Variations on any of these steps may provide a clue to the cause for postoperative symptoms, and also the hope that revisiting the operation may offer more success.

Once the old evaluation and operation has been reviewed, a new, thorough evaluation is begun. Because the anatomy has been altered by surgery, the preoperative tests no longer pertain, and the entire preoperative work-up must be undertaken, including EGD, 24-hour pH testing, esophageal manometery, and video esophagography [72].

EGD will demonstrate exposed suture material, residual hiatal hernia, and even the integrity of the fundoplication in a retroflexed angle. Barium esophagram will allow visualization of the anatomic defect. Esophageal manometry may identify if the fundoplication is too tight (LES too high) or too loose (LES too low). Esophageal body motility testing may identify previously missed or newly unmasked motor abnormalities such as achalasia, Nutcracker esophagus, or diffuse esophageal spasm. A 24-hour pH test can confirm or refute recurrent or persistent reflux as part of the postoperative symptom complex.

The choice of a laparoscopic open approach to redo surgery depends on the surgeon's experience. Multiple reports exist in successful laparoscopic revision of fundoplications in cases of failed antireflux surgery [73–75]. In either approach, the liver is densely adherent to the wrap, and requires meticulous dissection to avoid injury to the esophagus, stomach, or liver. The operative strategy should focus on any abnormalities demonstrated preoperatively, including recurrent hiatal hernia, existence of short esophagus, or a lack of short gastric division. The wrap should be taken down completely and the fundus returned to its usual anatomic position. Once the anatomy of the area has been exposed, the authors proceed as we do for first-time antireflux surgery.

Summary

Much progress has been made in the surgical management of gastroesophageal reflux disease. Early operations were plagued by hernia recurrence, gas bloat symptoms, and recurrence. The prospect of thoracotomy or laparotomy may have made patients and referring physicians reluctant to proceed with surgery. Thoughtful surgical research has led to better understanding of the mechanisms of reflux. Modifications based on this work have improved outcomes. The shorter, looser wrap is better tolerated than the original, and laparoscopic approaches have reduced recovery times while maintaining excellent results. The next era of treatment of acid reflux disorders will certainly build upon this work, continuing to fine-tune our approach to this widespread disorder.

References

[1] Deschamps C. Surgical treatment of gastroesophageal reflux disease. In: Jamieson GG, Duranceau A, editors. Gastroesophageal reflux. Philadelphia: WB Saunders; 1988. p. 122–57.

[2] Nissen R, Eine E, Einfat HE. Operation zur Beeinflussung der R defluxochtitis [Surgery to influence reflux esophagitis]. Schweiz Med Wochenschr 1956;86:590–2 [in German].

[3] Hill L, Thor K, Mercer DC. Surgery for hiatal hernia and esophagitis. In: Hill L, Kozarck R, McCallum R, editors. The esophagus, medical and surgical management. Philadelphia: WB Saunders; 1988. p. 90–138.

[4] Allison PR. Reflux oesophagitis, sliding hiatal hernia and anatomy of repair. Surg Gynecol Obstet 1951;92:419–31.

[5] Allison PR. Hiatus hernia; a 20-year retrospective survey. Ann Surg 1973;178:273–6.

[6] Baue J, Belsey RHR. The treatment of sliding hiatus hernia and reflux esophagitis by the Mark IV technique. Surgery 1967;62:396–406.

[7] Hill LD. An effective operation for hiatal hernia: an 8 year appraisal. Ann Surg 1967;166: 681–92.

[8] Castell OD. The esophagus. In: DeMeester TR, Stein HJ, Their SO, editors. The surgical treatment of gastroesophageal reflux disease. Boston: Little, Brown and Company; 1992. p. 579–625.

[9] Polk HC, Zeppa R. Hiatal hernia and esophagitis. A survey of indications for operation and technique and results of fundoplication. Ann Surg 1971;173:775–81.

[10] Rossetti M, Heill K. Fundoplication for the treatment of gastroesophageal reflux in hiatal hernia. World J Surg 1977;1:439–43.

[11] Bushkin FL, Neustein CL, Parker TH, et al. Nissen fundoplication for reflux peptic esophagitis. Ann Surg 1977;185:672–7.

[12] Nicholson DA, Nohl-Oser JC. Hiatus hernia: a comparison between two methods of fundoplication by evaluation of the long term results. J Thorac Cardiovasc Surg 1976;72: 938–43.

[13] Negre JB, Markkula HT, Keyrilainen O, et al. Nissen fundoplication: results at 10 year follow-up. Am J Surg 1983;146:635–7.

[14] Ellis FH, Crozier RE. Reflux control by fundoplication: a clinical and manometric assessment of the Nissen operation. Ann Thorac Surg 1984;38:387–92.

[15] Woodward ER, Thomas HF, McAlhany JC. Comparison of crural repair and Nissen fundoplication in the treatment of esophageal hiatus hernia with peptic esophagitis. Ann Surg 1971;173:782–92.

[16] Donahue PE, Bombeck PT. The modified Nissen fundoplication—reflux prevention without gas bloat. Review of Surgery 1977;11:15–27.

[17] Donahue PE, Samuelson S, Nulus LM, et al. The floppy Nissen fundoplication—effective long term control of pathologic reflux. Arch Surg 1985;120:663–7.

[18] Demeester TR, Bonavina L, Albertucci M. Nissen fundoplication for gastroesophageal reflux disease. Evaluation of primary repair in 100 consecutive patients. Ann Surg 1986;204: 9–20.

[19] Guarner V, Degollade JR, Tore NM. A new antireflux procedure at the esophagogastric junction: experimental and clinical evaluation. Arch Surg 1975;110:101–6.

[20] Menguy R. A modified fundoplication which preserves the ability to belch. Surgery 1978;84: 301–7.

[21] Thor K. The modified Toupet procedure. In: Hill L, Kozarck R, McCallum R, editors. The esophagus, medical and surgical management. Philadelphia: WB Saunders; 1988. p. 135–8.

[22] Lund RF, Wetscher GF, Raiser F, et al. Laparosocipic Toupet fundoplication for gastroesophageal reflux disease with poor esophageal body motility. J Gastrointest Surg 1997;1:301–8.

[23] Lim JK, Moisidis E, Munro WS, et al. Re-operation for failed anti-reflux surgery. Aust N Z J Surg 1996;66:731–3.

[24] Lindeboom MA, Ringers J, Straathof JW, et al. Effect of laparoscopic partial fundoplication on reflux mechanisms. Am J Gastroenterol 2003;98:29–34.

[25] Jobe BA, Wallace J, Hansen PD, et al. Evaluation of laparoscopic Toupet fundoplication as a primary repair for all patients with medically resistant gastroesophageal reflux. Surg Endosc 1997;11:1080–3.

[26] Horvath KD, Jobe BA, Herron DM, et al. Laparoscopic Toupet fundoplication is an inadequate procedure for patients with severe reflux disease. J Gastrointest Surg 1999;3: 583–91.

[27] Dallemagne B, Weerts JM, Jehaes C. Laparoscopic Nissen fundoplication: preliminary report. Surg Laparosc Endosc 1991;1:138–43.

[28] Cuschieri A, Hunter J, Wolfe B, et al. Multicenter evaluation of laparoscopic antireflux surgery. Preliminary report. Surg Endosc 1993;7:505–10.

[29] Peters JH, Heimbucher J, Kauer KH, et al. Clinical and physiologic comparison of laparoscopic and open Nissen fundoplication. J Am Coll Surg 1995;180:385–93.

[30] Hinder RA, Filipi CJ, Wetscher G, et al. Laparoscopic Nissen fundoplication is an effective treatment for gastroesophageal reflux disease. Ann Surg 1994;220:472–83.

[31] Jamieson GG, Watson DI, Britten-Jones R, et al. Laparoscopic Nissen fundoplication. Ann Surg 1994;220:137–45.

[32] Hunter JG, Trus TL, Branum GD, et al. A physiologic approach to laparoscopic fundoplication for gastroesophageal reflux disease. Ann Surg 1996;223:673–87.

[33] Gotley DC, Smithers BM, Rhodes M, et al. Laparoscopic Nissen fundoplication—200 consecutive cases. Gut 1996;38:487–91.

[34] Watson DI, Hamieson GG, Baigrie RJ, et al. Laparoscopic surgey for gastroesophageal reflux: beyond the learning curve. Br J Surg 1996;83:1284–7.

[35] Cattey RP, Henry LG, Bielfield MR. Laparoscopic Nissen fundoplication for gastroesoph-ageal reflux disease: clinical experience and outcome in first 100 patients. Surg Laparosc Endosc 1996;6:430–3.

[36] Nilsson G, Wenner J, Larsson S, et al. Randomized clinical trial of laparoscopic versus open fundoplication for gastroesophageal reflux. Br J Surg 2004;91:552–9.

[37] Ackroyd R, Watson DI, Majeed AW, et al. Randomized clinical trial of laparoscopic versus open fundoplication for gastroesophageal reflux disease. Br J Surg 2004;91:975–82.

[38] Chrysos E, Tsiaoussis J, Athanasakis E, et al. Laparoscopic versus open approach for Nissen fundoplication: a comparative study. Surg Endosc 2002;16:1679–84.

[39] Wenner J, Nilsson G, Oberg S, et al. Short-term outcome after laparoscopic and open 360-degree fundoplication: a prospective randomized clinical trial. Surg Endosc 2001;15:1124–8.

[40] Laine S, Rantala A, Gullichsen R, et al. Laparoscopic versus conventional Nissen fundoplication: a prospective randomized study. Surg Endosc 1997;11:441–4.

[41] Ritter MP, Peters JH, DeMeester TR, et al. Outcome after laparoscopic fundoplication is not dependent on a structurally defective lower esophageal sphincter. J Gastrointest Surg 1998;6:567–71.

[42] Johnson WE, Hagan JA, DeMeester TR, et al. Outcome of respiratory symptoms after antireflux surgery on patients with gastroesophageal reflux disease. Arch Surg 1996;131:489–92.

[43] Axelrod DA, Divi V, Ajluni MM, et al. Influence of functional bowel disease on outcome of surgical antireflux procedures. J Gastrointest Surg 2002;6:632–7.

[44] Raftopoulos Y, Papasavas P, Landreneau R, et al. Clinical outcome of laparoscopic antireflux surgery for patients with irriq1bowel syndorome. Surg Endosc 2004;18:655–9.

[45] Pellegrini C. Delayed gastric emptying in patients with abnormal gastroesophageal reflux. Ann Surg 2001;234:147–8.

[46] Blum AL, Tally NJ, O'Morain C, et al. Lack of effect of treating *Helicobacter pylori* infection in patients with nonulcer dyspepsia. Omeprazole plus clarithromycin and amoxicillin effect one year after treatment study group. N Engl J Med 1998;339:1875–81.

[47] Lundell LR, Myers JC, Jamieson GG. Delayed gastric emptying and its relationship to symptoms of "gas bloat" after antireflux surgery. Eur J Surg 1994;16:161–6.

[48] Greason KL, Miller LD, Deschamps C, et al. Effects of antireflux procedures on respiratory symptoms. Ann Thorac Surg 2002;73:381–5.

[49] Field SK, Gelfand GAJ, McFakken SD. The effects of antireflux surgery on asthmatics with gastroesophageal reflux. Chest 1999;116:766–74.

[50] Campos GM, Peters JH, DeMeester TR. Multivariate analysis of the factors predicting outcome after laparoscopic Nissen fundoplication. J Gastrointest Surg 1999;3:292–300.

[51] Jamison JR, Stein HJ, DeMeester TR. Ambulatory 24-hour esophageal pH monitoring: normal values, optimal thresholds specificity, sensitivity, and reproducibility. Am J Gastroenterol 1992;87:1102–11.

[52] Johnson LF, Demeester TR. Development of the 24 hour intraesophageal pH monitoring composite scoring system. J Clin Gastroenterol 1986;8:52–8.

[53] Stein HJ, DeMeester TR, Naspetti R. The three-dimensional lower esophageal sphincter pressure profile in gastroesophageal reflux disease. Ann Surg 1991;214:374.

[54] Pearson FG, Todd TR. Gastroplasty and fundoplication for complex reflux problems: long-term results. Ann Surg 1987;206:473–81.

[55] Hill LD, Gelfand M, Bauermeister D. Simplified management of reflux esophagitis with stricture. Ann Surg 1970;172:638–51.

[56] Swanstrom LL, Marcus DR, Galloway GQ. Laparoscopic Collis gastroplasty is the treatment of choice for the shortened esophagus. Am J Surg 1996;171:477–81.

[57] Johnson AB, Oddsdottir M, Hunter JG. Laparoscopic Collis gastroplasty and Nissen fundoplication: a new technique for the management of esophageal foreshortening. Surg Endosc 1998;12:1055–60.

[58] Awad ZT, Mittal SK, Roth TA. Esophageal shortening during the era of laparoscopic surgery. World J Surg 2001;25:558–61.

[59] Gastal OL, Hagen JA, Peters JH. Short esophagus: analysis of predictors and clinical implications. Arch Surg 1999;134:633–6.

[60] Hunter JG, Swanstrom LL, Waring JP. Dysphagia after laparoscopic antireflux surgery: the impact of operative technique. Ann Surg 1996;224:51–7.

[61] Pearson FG, Henderson RD. Long-term follow-up of peptic strictures managed by dilation, modified Collis gastroplasty and Belsey hiatus hernia repair. Surgery 1976;80:396–401.

[62] Stirling MC, Orringer MB. Continued assessment of the combined Collis-Nissen operation. Ann Thorac Surg 1989;47:224–30.

[63] Steichen FM. Abdominal approach to the Collis gastroplasty and Nissen fundoplication. Surg Gynecol Obstet 1986;162:372–4.

[64] Frantzides C, Madan AK, Carlson MA. A prospective, randomized trial of laparoscopic polytetrafluroethylene patch repair vs. simple cruroplasty for large hiatal hernia. Arch Surg 2002;137:649–53.

[65] Champion JK, McKernan JB. Hiatal size and risk of recurrence after laparoscopic fundoplication. Surg Endosc 1998;12:565–70.

[66] Granderath FA, Kamolz T, Schweiger UM. Laparoscopic refundoplication with prosthetic hiatal closure for recurrent hiatal hernia after primary failed antireflux surgery. Arch Surg 2003;138:902–7.

[67] Perdikis G, Hinder RA, Wetscher GJ. Nissen fundoplication for gastroesophageal reflux disease: laparoscopic Nissen fundoplication—technique and results. Dis Esophagus 1996;9:272–7.

[68] Eubanks TR, Omelanczuk P, Richards C, et al. Outcomes of laparoscopic antireflux procedures. Am J Surg 2000;179:391–5.

[69] Hinder RA, Klingler PJ, Perdikis G, et al. Management of the failed antireflux operation. Surg Clin North Am 1997;77:1083–97.

[70] Dallemagne B, Weerts JM, Jehaes C, et al. Causes of failures of laparoscopic antireflux operations. Surg Endosc 1996;10(3):305–10.

[71] Perez AR, Moncure AC, Rattner DW. Obesity is a major cause of failure for both transabdominal and transthorcic antireflux operations. Presented at the 100th Annual Meeting of the American Gastroenterological Association. Chicago, Illinois, May 14–19, 2005.

[72] Horgan S, Pohl D, Bogetti D, et al. Failed antireflux surgery: what have we learned from reoperations? Arch Surg 1999;134(8):809–15.

[73] Curet MJ, Josloff RK, Schoeb O, et al. Laparoscopic reoperation for failed antireflux procedures. Arch Surg 1999;134:559–63.

[74] O'Reilly M, Mullins S, Reddick EJ. Laparoscopic management of failed antireflux surgery. Surg Laparosc Endosc Percutan Tech 1997;7:90–3.

[75] Granderth FA, Kamolz T, Schwiger UM, et al. Is laparoscopic refundoplication feasible in patients with failed primary open antireflux surgery? Surg Endosc 2002;16:381–5.

ELSEVIER
SAUNDERS

SURGICAL
CLINICS OF
NORTH AMERICA

Surg Clin N Am 85 (2005) 949–965

Endoscopic Therapy for Gastroesophageal Reflux Disease

Richard I. Rothstein, MD*, Andrew C. Dukowicz, MD

Section of Gastroenterology and Hepatology, Dartmouth Medical School, Dartmouth Hitchcock Medical Center, One Medical Center Drive, Lebanon, NH 03756, USA

Gastroesophageal reflux disease (GERD) is a common chronic gastro-intestinal disorder that produces symptoms in at least 19 million individuals annually, and creates a direct cost of over 10 billion dollars in the United States alone [1]. Goals of antireflux therapy should be directed toward symptom relief, long-term remission, healing of esophagitis, and prevention of complications of GERD. Treatments for GERD have evolved over time, and have mainly involved suppression or neutralization of stomach acid, or surgical manipulation of the stomach anatomy to enhance the antireflux barrier at the gastroesophageal junction (GEJ). Medical therapy directed at acid suppression with proton pump inhibitors (PPIs) has been shown to be safe and effective [2]; however, PPIs often incompletely relieve symptoms of heartburn, and frequently require daily dosing and dose escalation, which may be undesirable from a financial and quality-of-life (QOL) perspective.

Surgical therapy, most commonly with a laparoscopic fundoplication, is an option for patients who have either an inadequate response to medical therapy or a desire to be free of chronic medication use. The Nissen fundoplication has been shown to be about 90% effective for control of symptoms; however, it has been reported that up to half of patients required medications postoperatively for control of symptoms over a 10-year follow-up [3,4]. Drawbacks of the surgical approach remain, and include the prolonged recovery time (usually 1 day of hospitalization and up to 3 weeks of postoperative recovery, with restrictions on diet and exercise) and the development of new postoperative symptoms. Some series have reported that between 4% to 19% of patients can experience new symptoms of dysphagia, bloating, diarrhea, constipation, or abdominal pain postoperatively [5,6].

---

* Corresponding author.
 E-mail address: richard.i.rothstein@hitchcock.org (R.I. Rothstein).

0039-6109/05/$ - see front matter © 2005 Elsevier Inc. All rights reserved.
doi:10.1016/j.suc.2005.06.003

Both forms of GERD therapy come at a significant cost. For medical treatment, the long-term financial cost over many years of therapy is considerable, whereas the financial burden remains high up front for surgical intervention. Cost-efficacy models generally favor surgical treatment; however, they may not always factor in the costs of postoperative complications and future surgical interventions [7].

Within the last 15 years, novel endoscopic therapies have been developed as an additional option for patients who have GERD. These approaches can provide long-term relief of GERD, or can be used to "bridge" patients to future therapy, because undergoing treatment does not preclude one from future medical or surgical therapy. Thus far, there have been three separate approaches to endoscopic therapy:

1) Plication/sewing techniques—endoscopic plication (either full-thickness or submucosal) at the GEJ and gastric cardia
2) Radiofrequency thermal therapy delivered to the lower esophageal sphincter (LES)
3) Injection/implantation of a biopolymer into the region of the LES

These therapies continue to be an active source of research and investigation. Although they are undergoing rapid development, there are only a few peer-reviewed articles detailing original studies with short-term follow-up. Future success in this arena will depend on sham-controlled trials, long-term outcome studies, and cost-effectiveness analyses. The goal of this article is to describe available endoscopic therapies, discuss their effectiveness and duration of response, and review their failures and complications.

Plication/sewing techniques

The first endoscopic suturing system was developed in the mid-1980s [8] and has undergone several subsequent modifications that allow the endoscopist to place sutures into the gastric cardia, thereby augmenting the barrier effect of the GEJ. Two such devices have gained Food and Drug Administration (FDA) approval for antireflux therapy. The Bard Endo-Cinch system (Bard Endoscopic Technologies, Billerica, Massachusetts) uses a disposable sewing capsule that is attached to the distal end of a gastroscope to place sutures into the submucosa. The NDO Plicator (NDO Surgical, Mansfield, Massachusetts) is a reusable instrument that fits over a gastroscope and creates a full-thickness serosa-to-serosa apposition of the proximal gastric cardia. Other devices have been created, including the Wilson-Cook Endoscopic Suturing Device (ESD) (Wilson-Cook Medical, Winston-Salem, North Carolina) and the Syntheon Anti-Reflux Device (ARD) (Syntheon/ID, Miami, Florida). The Wilson-Cook ESD, modified from laparoscopic sewing instruments, was used in a small number of individuals following FDA approval; however, no prospective or controlled trials were ever reported. The company has now removed this device from commercial availability. The Syntheon ARD plicator initial trial is nearing completion, and a follow-up sham-controlled study is planned for this full-thickness plicating device.

Bard EndoCinch

The Bard EndoCinch system was the first endoscopic sewing and plication instrument created, and to date over 5000 clinical procedures have been performed worldwide using the device. It consists of a sewing capsule that is attached to the distal end of a gastroscope. The capsule has a hollow chamber through which esophageal tissue can be suctioned. A handle mounted to the biopsy port on the gastroscope then drives a hollow-core needle containing the suture material through the tissue to create a stitch through the submucosa. A second gastroscope must be used to fasten the ends of the sutures together.

Procedure

The procedure is done in the outpatient setting, most often using conscious sedation. After routine upper endoscopy is performed, an overtube is loaded onto a 42 or 45 French Savary-type esophageal dilator and advanced over a guidewire. The suturing capsule is attached to a second gastroscope and advanced via the overtube to the GEJ. The site to be sutured is identified (usually 1 cm distal to the z-line marking the squamo-columnar junction), and suction is applied to draw tissue into the capsule. The needle is advanced through the suctioned tissue, delivering a t-tag attached to the 3-0 monofilament into the cap of the device, and suction is released. The sewing capsule is withdrawn through the overtube, reloaded, and the stitching process repeated, with the second targeted area being about 1 centimeter apart from the initial one. The sewing endoscope is then removed from the overtube, and the two suture ends are available for fastening together to form the gastric pleat. The original technique required multiple passes of the second endoscope, because six half-hitches were hand-tied and pushed to the mucosal surface with a knot-pusher; however, the current technique uses a cinching/cutting catheter placed through the second endoscope, into which the suture ends are back-loaded. The scope and cinching catheter are guided to the gastric surface using the sutures as a "rail." A peg-and-ring fastener is deployed, cinching together the suture at the level of the stomach surface, and the suture ends are cut by actuating the catheter handle. The new technique can substantially reduce the time to complete a plication from about 15 minutes for each one to 5 or 10 minutes.

Preclinical data

Preclinical data showed promise for the EndoCinch device, and suggested some mechanisms of action. In a study of endoscopic gastroplasty in dogs

[9], the plication procedure produced a significant increase in lower esophageal sphincter pressure (LESP)—13.3 versus 4.6 mm Hg; and gastric yield pressure—19 versus 10 mm Hg. The yield pressure of the gastric cardia in this study, measured with an attached manometry catheter, was determined in vivo, with the endoscope in retroflexion observing the point at which the cardia opened during continuous air insufflation in response to increased intragastric pressure. Another study using a porcine model [10] showed a similar augmentation in LESP postgastroplasty, and additionally was found to reduce the median time pH was less than 4 from 9.3% to 0.2% of the time postprocedure.

Clinical data

The majority of early clinical trials for the EndoCinch device remain in abstract form; however, a pivotal multicenter trial was published in 2001 [11] and provided data for the FDA approval of the device for treatment of GERD. The trial suggested that endoscopic gastric plication is a safe procedure and, at a 6-month follow-up, that two thirds of patients undergoing the procedure were successfully treated. The inclusion criteria included three or more episodes of heartburn per week when off antisecretory medications, successful response to and reliance upon antisecretory medications for GERD, and abnormal acid reflux (evidenced by a pH <4 for more than 4% of the time) on ambulatory pH monitoring. Exclusion criteria included dysphagia, Grade II Savary-Miller erosive esophagitis while on medications, body mass index (BMI) greater than 40 kg/m^2, GERD refractory to PPIs, and a hiatal hernia greater than 2 cm in length.

Treatment success was defined as a decrease in the heartburn severity score by 50%, in addition to a reduction in the use of antireflux medications to fewer than four doses per month. Subjects were randomized to either linear or circumferential suture plication, and underwent endoscopy, esophageal manometry, ambulatory pH monitoring, symptoms severity scoring, and QOL assessments before and after endoscopic therapy. Sixty-four patients were enrolled in the trial. Thirty-three patients (52%) underwent endoscopic gastroplication with a linear configuration, and 31 patients (48%) underwent a circumferential plication. There was no difference in outcomes between the linear and circumferential groups. Mean heartburn scores (calculated by multiplying the heartburn severity score by the frequency score) fell from a preprocedure score of 62.7 to mean scores of 16.7 and 17 at 3 and 6 months postprocedure, respectively. In addition, regurgitation scores significantly improved during the same time interval. Although there was no change in LES pressure pre- and postprocedure, the percent total time pH was less than 4, total number of reflux episodes, and the percent upright time pH was less than 4 were all significantly improved at the 6-month follow-up, and one third of subjects had their pH scores normalized. Most importantly, QOL scores were improved for social functioning and bodily pain, and 62% of patient achieved predefined treatment success by using fewer than four doses of antireflux medications per month. Adverse events included pharyngitis (31%), vomiting (14%), and abdominal or chest pain (14%–16%). Oxygen desaturation occurred during the procedure in 4 patients. There were two episodes of minor mucosal tears that were felt to be due to the use of a large overtube, and 1 patient experienced a suture microperforation that was treated conservatively with intravenous antibiotics and brief hospitalization.

Since this initial trial, 2-year follow-up data on a subset (33 patients) of the original cohort have been reported in abstract form [12]. These patients continued to report a significant improvement in their heartburn severity and frequency; however, the frequency of regurgitation was no longer significantly improved. Finally, 25% of patients were off all antisecretory medications, 28% were on less than half of their initial medication doses, 41% were on full-dose medications, and 6% had undergone laparoscopic Nissen fundoplication. A report with 2-year follow-up of 85 patients from five centers involved in an early treatment experience [13] showed that 51% of patients had no or only occasional GERD symptoms, and 56% were completely off PPIs or taking less than one dose per week. Economic analysis in that study showed a reduction in the mean annual medication cost from $2424 per year preprocedure to $860 per year postprocedure [13].

More recently, a randomized, blinded, sham-controlled single-institution EndoCinch study has been reported [14]. Subjects were more than 18 years old, had symptomatic heartburn at least 3 to 5 days a week, were dependent upon acid-suppressive medications for symptom control, and had abnormal acid exposure on pH study, a normal esophageal manometry, and a hiatal hernia 3 cm or less. Thirty-four subjects were enrolled; 17 underwent four circumferential gastric plications and 17 underwent a sham operation designed to mimic the actual gastroplication in every way except placement of sutures. At 3-month follow-up, there was a significant difference in heartburn frequency score (gastric plication 69% versus sham 31%, $P = 0.03$), but no significant difference in heartburn severity, regurgitation, or bothersome score between the two groups. Significantly more patients who underwent gastric plication were able to discontinue daily acid-suppressing medications compared with shams (75% versus 25%, $P = 0.01$); however there was no difference found between the two groups when comparing discontinuation of all antisecretory medications. Esophageal acid exposure significantly improved in the treatment group, but only normalized in 2 subjects (12.5%).

The Bard EndoCinch has been directly compared with laparoscopic Nissen fundoplication in a small study setting [15]. Sixteen patients underwent endoscopic therapy and were compared with 18 age-matched controls who underwent surgical treatment. The mean procedure time (52 versus 116 minutes) and mean length of hospital stay (0.05 versus 3.3 days) favored those patients undergoing endoscopic therapy. Symptom scores, PPI requirement, and QOL scores improved significantly in both groups; however the surgical group showed greater control of esophageal acid exposure.

NDO Plicator

The NDO Plicator differs from the Bard EndoCinch by creating a full-thickness, serosa-to-serosa apposition of the proximal cardia. Originally placed via an overtube, the latest version of the plicator can be passed via a guidewire, and contains a channel into which a small 5.9-mm pediatric gastroscope can be passed to allow direct visualization of the cardia while the plication is created. The NDO device operator positions, opens, and closes the arms of the instrument via knob controls on the instrument handle. Through the center of the instrument, a stainless steel corkscrew tissue retractor is used to engage an area of the cardia just beneath the GEJ, pulling it between the instrument arms to be plicated. The current system incorporates an implant (pretied 2-0 polypropylene with polytetrafluroethylene bolters) as a single-use cartridge that is loaded into the arms of the plicator.

Procedure

After routine upper endoscopy under conscious sedation, a guidewire is passed and left in the distal stomach. After withdrawing the gastroscope, the NDO Plicator can be directly passed over the guidewire. After passage of the Plicator, a small-caliber gastroscope can be passed through the center of the Plicator and retroflexed upon reaching the stomach to visualize the site of plication. The tissue retractor is then inserted deep in the tissue of the gastric cardia, usually within 1 cm from the GEJ. This area is pulled between the instrument arms as they are closed. Upon closing the arms of the device, a pretied monofilament suture implant is deployed to fix the tissue together. After disengaging the tissue retractor, the endoscope and NDO device are straightened and removed from the patient.

Preclinical data

Preclinical studies have been reported in live miniswine as well as ex vivo porcine stomachs to evaluate the safety of the procedure and monitor the effectiveness of the full-thickness plication [16]. In the safety part of the study, 11 miniswine underwent full-thickness plication, then a period of observation from 0 to 12 weeks. They underwent repeat endoscopy before sacrifice—there were no signs of tissue damage or trauma noted during either endoscopy or examination of the excised stomach. Studies designed to measure the gastric yield pressure showed an increase up to eightfold without a significant change in esophageal diameter.

Clinical data

An initial pilot study involved six patients who had symptomatic reflux requiring maintenance PPI therapy [17]. All patients underwent a full-thickness plication in the gastric cardia and were followed clinically (symptoms and medication use), endoscopically, and via 24-hour pH/manometry at 3, 6, and 12 months postprocedure. The mean procedure time was 21 minutes. At 6 months postprocedure, five of the six patients were off acid-suppressive medications, and at 12 months mean symptom score and QOL measurements were improved over 75%. Both 24-hour pH and total number of reflux episodes improved in the majority of patients, and no significant change in esophageal manometry was noted. Follow-up endoscopy confirmed that the original plications remained intact at the 1-year check.

The NDO Plicator has received recent FDA approval for antireflux therapy after a recent US multicenter trial [18]. The study involved 64 GERD patients at seven participating centers. These patients had heartburn or regurgitation requiring acid-suppressive medications for more than 6 months, an abnormal pH study, and normal esophageal peristalsis on manometry. Patients who had hiatal hernia greater than 2 cm, Grade III or greater esophagitis, or Barrett's epithelium were excluded. All patients underwent a single full-thickness plication (mean time of procedure 17.2 minutes) and were asked to discontinue all antireflux medications by 7 days postprocedure. At 6-month follow-up, GERD QOL scores improved by 67%, and 74% of patients had discontinued their previous daily PPI use. PH probe testing showed normalization of distal esophageal acid exposure in 29%, similar to other endoscopic modalities. There was no noted change in LESP or other parameters of esophageal motility. Additional follow-up showed that 70% of patients were still off their PPIs at 12 months postprocedure. Adverse events after the plication procedure included pharyngitis (41%), abdominal pain (20%), chest pain (17%), gastrointestinal (GI) disorder (17%), eructation (14%), dysphagia (11%), and nausea (6%). Serious adverse events occurred in 6 patients. Dyspnea occurred in 2 patients shortly after placement of the overtube (the multicenter trial was done with the earlier version of the NDO device)—1 patient required endotracheal intubation for airway compromise. Both patients subsequently completed the procedure under propofol. Another patient developed a spontaneous pneumothorax that resolved with conservative treatment. Two patients developed pneumoperitoneum—one underwent an exploratory laparotomy (which did not reveal a perforation); the other was noted to have a small gastric perforation during the procedure, and was treated with endoclip closure and a course of antibiotics with no clinical sequelae. There have been subsequent modifications to the device (including covering the retractable arms in a flexible membrane to decrease the risk of tissue trauma), and the current instrument version no longer requires an overtube. This device evolution will likely reduce the number of safety issues seen in the initial trial.

A multicenter, international, sham-controlled study is currently underway. There has not yet been a direct comparison of the NDO device with surgical fundoplication.

In addition to these trials, further investigation with single verses multiple suture implants would be helpful to identify the ideal location, number, and placement of the plications.

Radiofrequency thermal therapy

Another endoscopic approach involves the delivery of low-power, temperature-controlled radiofrequency (RF) energy to the GEJ, more specifically to the muscularis propria. RF energy ablation has been used in a number of disease settings, including cardiac arrhythmias, sleep-disordered breathing, joint capsule laxity, solid organ (including hepatic) tumors, and benign prostate hypertrophy. Whereas rapid heating of tissue causes desiccation, raising the tissue temperature in a controlled manner allows propagation of heat and formation of controlled lesions. In endoscopic therapy for GERD, RF energy is thought to enhance LES function by reducing the frequency of transient LES relaxations, and by augmenting the barrier effect of the LES with increased LES pressure after the procedure [19,20]. Since being approved by the FDA in 2000, more than 5000 patients have received RF thermal therapy via the Stretta System (Curon Medical, Inc., Sunnyvale, California). The Stretta system consists of a control unit that monitors tissue temperature and impedance, and disposable single-use RF catheters that contain four deployable needles. Thermocouples on the tip and base of the needles permit the monitoring of energy delivery to deeper tissues and to the surface epithelium. The needles can function independently, with an automatic shutoff if desired temperatures are exceeded.

Procedure

After routine upper endoscopy is done with the goal of identifying landmarks and determining the presence of a hiatal hernia greater than 3 cm or Barrett's esophagus (which would make the procedure contraindicated), a guidewire is fed through the gastroscope to the distal stomach. After removal of the gastroscope, the Stretta treatment catheter is passed over the guidewire and positioned at the GEJ. The first set or "ring" of thermal lesions is created approximately 1 cm above the GEJ. Each set is comprised of two deployments of the catheter while it is rotated 45° between deployments. Currently, the RF energy is delivered to each electrode for 60 seconds. The full Stretta procedure involves placing four antegrade rings from 1 cm above the GEJ to just below the squamocolumnar junction in .5 cm increments, as well as two retrograde rings in the gastric cardia. Due to the tendency of the catheter to migrate distally during the procedure, it is suggested to pass an endoscope after placement of the first two rings in order to check the position and to adjust accordingly. The procedure generally takes 45 to 55 minutes to complete.

Preclinical data

Using a porcine model for GERD that incorporated botulinum toxin to relax the LES, the Stretta procedure was shown to augment LES pressure and gastric yield pressure [21]. One week after receiving 100 U of botulinum toxin into the LES, 20 pigs were randomized to control (n = 7) or treatment with RF energy (n = 13). The group receiving the RF energy treatment had a mean increase in LES pressure of 21% at 8 weeks post-treatment, compared with a 27% drop in LES pressure at 9 weeks in the control group. Additionally, the group treated with RF energy had a 75% augmentation in gastric yield pressure. Again using a porcine model, additional investigation [22] showed an increase in muscle thickness of the LES via endoscopic ultrasound (EUS) at 1 week post-RF energy delivery. This finding was corroborated on histology specimens.

Clinical data

In the initial uncontrolled Stretta multicenter trials, enrolled patients included those who had symptomatic GERD with some benefit from antireflux medications. Exclusion criteria included hiatal hernia greater than 2 cm, greater than grade 2 esophagitis, Barrett's metaplasia, severe dysphagia, previous esophageal or gastric surgery, collagen vascular disease, or significant medical comorbidities. These study patients (47 at 6 months, 94 at 12 months) showed a significant improvement in GERD-related study parameters, including median heartburn score (improved from 4 to 1), median GERD score (27 to 9), PPI requirement (88% to 30%), and overall patient satisfaction (from 1 to 4) [23,24]. In addition, distal esophageal acid exposure improved significantly from 10.2% to 6.4%. There was not a significant increase in LES pressure, however, and the percentage of patients who had esophagitis did not significantly improve at 6 months. The procedure was well-tolerated, with 10 adverse events (representing 8.6% of the study population). All complications were acute and self-limited, and included superficial mucosal injury, fever, chest discomfort, transient dysphagia, sedation-related hypotension, and topical anesthesia allergy (all complications occurred in 2.6% or less of the study population).

In an effort to correlate physiologic response with symptomatic benefit, a recent subgroup analysis comparing "responders" and "nonresponders" (determined based on whether their distal esophageal acid exposure time improved) was performed [25]. A correlation was noted between an improvement in distal esophageal acid exposure and GERD health-related QOL and heartburn severity.

As noted before, the Stretta procedure has been performed on over 5000 patients since its approval by the FDA in 2000. The largest published collection of treated patients involves a registry of 558 patients from 33 separate institutions, with a mean follow-up of 8 months [26]. Most patients went from daily or twice-daily PPI use to no medication use or antacids use as needed. Additionally, patients showed a significant improvement in satisfactory control of their GERD symptoms (from 26% baseline on medications to 77% after Stretta) as well as a high degree of overall satisfaction.

Unfortunately, since its commercial release, there have been several reports of perforations and three deaths associated with the Stretta procedure. These all occurred early after the marketing release, and no serious complications have been reported more recently.

A recently published randomized, double-blinded, sham-controlled trial [27] displayed the superiority of the Stretta procedure in 35 patients who underwent the procedure compared with 29 patients who received a sham procedure. Patients undergoing the sham procedure underwent a similar preparation, conscious sedation, and routine upper endoscopy. The sham procedure employed a similar catheter with an identical feel and characteristics (except that no needles were deployed), and the investigators used a dialog similar to actual treatment during the procedure. After 6 months of follow-up, if still symptomatic, the sham patients were offered the actual procedure. During the 6-month trial, patients undergoing the Stretta procedure noted significantly fewer daily heartburn symptoms (61% versus 33%) and overall improved GERD QOL scores (61% noted >50% improvement compared with 30% in sham patients). Improvement in symptoms was noted to be persistent at 12-month follow-up; however, there was no difference found between groups in daily medication use or esophageal acid exposure times at 6 months. The study authors concluded that the symptomatic benefit of the procedure was not due to a sham effect. Additionally, this finding emphasizes the fact that endoscopic therapy may be best directed at individuals who have nonerosive reflux (most patients who have GERD), because a reliable decrease in esophageal acid exposure to heal erosive esophagitis has not been demonstrated.

Injection/implantation techniques

Implantation of a biopolymer into the LES in an effort to increase the antireflux barrier of the muscle has been around since the 1980s. An initial animal model using Teflon paste and bovine collagen injected into the distal esophagus of dogs that were surgically altered to have GERD (via LES myotomy and sphincterotomy) showed promise, with seven of the nine dogs showing improvement in some reflux parameters after the procedure [28]. An initial pilot trial was performed in 10 humans who had medically intractable symptoms [29]. These patients underwent injection into four quadrants above the squamocolumnar junction. Initially there was a 50% to 75% reduction in reflux symptoms and medication usage, as well as a significant improvement in esophageal acid exposure. At 12 month follow-up, however, most patients had a return to their baseline reflux symptoms and medication use. Follow-up endoscopy showed resorption of the implant material. The authors concluded that the initial trial was promising, but that the ideal implantation material was yet to be found.

Since then, other materials have been investigated. A small study used polymethylmethacrylate (PMMA, Plexiglas) injected into the LES of 10 patients who had GERD requiring PPIs and abnormal esophageal acid exposure times [30]. At 6- and 14.5-month follow-up, the patients showed significant improvement in GERD symptom scores and distal esophageal acid exposure times compared with baseline values. Seven of the 10 patients were off antireflux medications. Additionally, the procedure was well-tolerated, with 2 patients experiencing transient chest pain during the procedure. Finally, EUS performed at 6 months documented that PMMA microspheres were found scattered around the submucosa and small amounts were seen in the muscular layer. Although promising, no further trials have been performed with PMMA.

Enteryx

Enteryx (Boston Scientific, Natick, Massachusetts) is an injectable biocompatible solution consisting of 8% ethylene vinyl alcohol (EVOH) copolymer mixed in dimethyl sulfoxide (DMSO). When initially injected into the LES, the solution interacts with the surrounding fluid to become an inert spongy solid mass. The solution is mixed with micronized tantalum powder to provide radio opaque contrast during fluoroscopy.

Procedure

After routine upper endoscopy, a 23 gauge, 4-mm long catheter is flushed with DMSO, then filled with Enteryx solution, and advanced through the endoscope's accessory channel. The solution is injected at the squamocolumnar junction by advancing the needle into the LES muscle. The injection is made under fluoroscopic and endoscopic visualization to prevent submucosal or transmural injection of the solution. The solution is injected very slowly (rapid injection can generate heat), about 1 mL/min, and 1 to 2 mL is placed in four quadrants around the LES. After injecting the Enteryx, the needle is left in the injection site for 20 seconds thereafter to allow the solution to solidify and prevent leakage. The procedure is done in the outpatient setting, and patients can be expected to experience some postprocedure discomfort that is typically amenable to oral analgesics. Also, because some patients may note transient dysphagia postprocedure, they are instructed to stay on a soft mechanical diet for a few days thereafter. They are asked to wean their PPI use over the subsequent 1 to 2 weeks. If the patient does not get adequate control of symptoms after the first treatment, the implantation can be repeated—25% of patients in the first pilot study were retreated. Of note, in contrast to some of the other endoscopic therapies for GERD, the procedure is not reversible.

Preclinical data

Using a porcine model, Enteryx was shown to be safe and effective [31]. Implantation in 15 animals demonstrated a significant increase in gastric yield pressure, although sphincter length and resting pressure were unaffected. The animals were observed for up to 12 months and did not appear to develop any repercussions of the implantation—they tolerated the implantation well, ate well, and gained weight normally.

Clinical data

The initial pilot study for Enteryx was conducted in 15 patients who had GERD requiring continuous antisecretory therapy with PPIs [32]. The investigators achieved their primary objective by demonstrating the safety of the procedure (no procedural complications, 8 patients who had mild chest discomfort that resolved within 3 days, 1 patient who had mild transient dysphagia), increased LES pressure (seen at 1 and 6 months postprocedure), and stability of the injected biopolymer (9/15 patients had 50% of the injected material in place at 6 months). As a secondary end point, improvement of heartburn score was found in 14 of 15 patients at 1 month, and 13 of 15 patients at 6 months. Two patients had resumed full-dose PPI, whereas 2 other patients were using omeprazole on an as-needed basis.

More recently, data from the international multicenter, prospective, nonrandomized trial were published with follow-up data over a 12-month period [33,34]. The primary objective was assessment of PPI use at 6- and 12-month follow-up. Secondary objectives included analysis of GERD symptom scores, QOL, esophageal acid exposures, and manometric measurements after treatment. The study involved 85 patients who had symptoms of GERD responsive to PPIs, and who had GERD health–related QOL scores lower than 11 while on PPIs and greater than 20 off medications. In addition, they were required to have prolonged esophageal acid exposure times, with pH probe yielding pH of 4 or less more than 5% of the total time. Exclusion criteria included hiatal hernia greater than 3 cm, Barrett's esophagus, grade 3 or 4 esophagitis, or esophageal motility disorders. The study met the primary objective, with 74% of patients off all PPIs at 6 months, and 70% at 12 months. In addition, there was a significant improvement in mean esophageal acid exposure at both time intervals postprocedure, with normalization in about one third. Finally, heartburn and regurgitation symptom scores improved significantly as well. The mean procedure time was 34 minutes. The procedure was well-tolerated, with the majority of patients noting transient mild to moderate chest discomfort postprocedure lasting less than 2 weeks (most resolving within 5–7 days). Seventeen patients (20%) noted transient dysphagia postprocedure, most resolving within 2 weeks and all resolving within 12 weeks. Based on this trial, the Enteryx procedure was approved by the FDA in April, 2003, and over 3000 individuals have been treated worldwide. Post-marketing data have revealed one death that was attributable to the injection of Enteryx. Currently, both a post-marketing long-term follow-up analysis and a multicenter, randomized, sham-controlled trial are underway.

Gatekeeper

The Gatekeeper system (Medtronic, Minneapolis, Minnesota) is another form of implantation therapy for GERD, and incorporates the submucosal placement of a polyacrylonitrile-based hydrogel (HYPAN) bioprosthesis into the area of the LES. The procedure involves the use of a 16-mm diameter overtube, through which a standard or pediatric endoscope is passed.

Procedure

After routine endoscopy with careful notation of landmarks, a guidewire is advanced to the distal stomach, and the Gatekeeper overtube is advanced to the squamocolumnar junction. Suction is applied to the mucosa and submucosa to stabilize the overtube, and using a flexible sclerotherapy-type needle, saline is injected to create a submucosal pocket. After removal of the injection needle, a trocar is passed to pierce the saline collection, and then the hydrogel implant is placed into the submucosal pocket via a pushrod. The hydrogel implants are 20×1 mm in size, and resemble pieces of pencil lead. After implantation they swell to approximately 10 mm in diameter. Typically four to six implants are placed in a single session, and are positioned in a radial fashion by rotating the overtube (only one pass of the overtube and endoscope is needed). The implantation of the first prosthesis takes approximately 15 minutes, then 5 minutes each is required for each subsequent implant. One advantage of the procedure is its reversibility—if needed, the hydrogel implants can be excised using a needle knife, and extracted with gentle suction into a variceal banding "cap" attached to the distal end of a gastroscope.

Preclinical data

A recent study demonstrated the ease of learning the Gatekeeper technique and long-term retention of the implanted hydrogel prostesis [35]. Using farm pigs or miniswine, 98% of delivery attempts were successful. In addition, 88% of the implants were retained at 6 months, and 18 of 19 were retained at 3 years. Finally, the implants were demonstrated to be easily removable, successfully being removed in four of four attempts. Extraction via endoscopy generally took approximately 5 minutes per implant.

Clinical data

The initial pilot study using Gatekeeper involved 10 patients who had known GERD responsive to PPI therapy [36]. The implants were successfully placed in 97% of attempts, and the mean procedure time was approximately 22 minutes. At 1 and 6 months follow-up, these patients noted improved heartburn symptoms scores and improved esophageal acid exposure. In addition, 7 of 9 patients had significantly decreased their medication usage (4 were off medications, and 3 reduced their PPI use by >50%). Only one adverse event was reported—postprandial nausea starting 1 week after implantation. The patient's symptoms resolved after removal of the implants.

Recently published pooled data from two prospective, nonrandomized European multicenter trials further studied the safety and effectiveness of the Gatekeeper system [37]. Sixty-eight patients who had heartburn and regurgitation and abnormal esophageal acid exposure on pH probe underwent treatment with up to six prostheses placed (mean 4.3 prostheses per procedure). At 1- and 6-month follow-up, 80.4% and 70.4% of the implants were retained, respectively. In addition, esophageal acid exposure times improved (from time with pH <4.0 decreasing from 9.1% to 6.1%) and median LES pressure was increased (from 8.8 mmHg at baseline to 13.8 mmHg at 6 months). Finally, median GERD heartburn-related QOL scores improved significantly in patients no longer using PPIs. There were two adverse events during the trial—one pharyngeal perforation caused by a malfunction of the overtube that has since been redesigned. The patient recovered well after close observation and antibiotic therapy. The other adverse effect was postprandial nausea in 1 patient that resolved with removal of the prosthesis.

Of note, an international, multicenter, randomized, sham-controlled trial to evaluate the Gatekeeper system is nearing completion and its results are anticipated soon.

Summary

The initial outcomes for the endoscopic treatments for GERD have been published, although much remains to be learned from randomized-controlled trials that are underway or recently concluded. All of the techniques will be studied in a sham-controlled protocol to understand the real effect of treatment, because in studies to date the sham effect ranges from 30% to 41%. It is important to note that the results presented from the initial clinical trials are from the investigators' learning curve experience, and it is anticipated that additional experience will provide better results.

In general, for all of the treatments, about 67% to 75% of treated subjects who have mild GERD will have significant symptom improvement and will be able to discontinue all antisecretory treatment for up to 12 months. Longer-term follow-up shows a declining effect of treatment, with individuals returning to PPI use, and we await the publication of 2- to 5-year follow-up to know the true durability of these therapies. The endoscopic treatments only normalize the distal esophageal daily acid exposure for about one third of patients, although most significantly trend toward normal following treatment. It is possible that improvements in technique or instrumentation may augment this outcome. The endoscopic treatments are mainly quite safe and easy to perform in the outpatient setting; however, with over 10,000 cases now performed, there have been some serious adverse events reported, including several perforations, hemorrhage requiring trans-fusion, and four procedure-related deaths occurring during the initial expe-rience of the treating clinicians. Education, training, and experience will be the means to minimize any untoward outcomes and provide a pathway to credentialing that will be needed.

We do not yet know the ideal treatment nor the ideal candidates for endoscopic GERD therapy. It is possible and likely that the fairly minimal interventions with these novel techniques, done for approval in the initial FDA safety trials, do not effect enough change in GERD pathophysiology. We do not know the optimum location, position, or number of stitches, pleats, RF treatments, implants or injections to effect a more durable, successful clinical outcome. The future will bring additional refinements in instrument design and procedural techniques, and the role of endoscopic GERD treatment is still being defined. Additional devices for GERD treatment are now in evolution. It is possible that these therapies will be valuable not only as treatments to substitute for long-term medical therapy for the patient who has mildly symptomatic GERD, but may also allow medical therapy to be successful when they are employed as adjuncts to ongoing pharmacological treatment. They may be useful in patients who have previously undergone a surgical fundoplication that no longer controls acid-related symptoms. They may have a role in treating the extra-esophageal symptoms of GERD, and this needs further study. It is early in the development of these novel approaches to GERD treatment, and the next few years will yield much additional study to help us identify their role in the management of our patients.

References

[1] Sandler RS, Everhart JE, Donowitz M, et al. The burden of selected digestive diseases in the United States. Gastroenterology 2002;122:1500–11.

[2] Klinkenberg-Knol EC, Nelis F, Dent J, et al. Long-tern omeprazole treatment in resistant gastro-esophageal reflux disease: efficacy, safety, and influence on gastric mucosa. Gastroenterology 2000;118:661–9.

[3] Lundell L, Miettinen P, Myrvold HE, et al. Long-term outcome of medical and surgical therapies for gastroesophageal reflux disease: follow-up of a randomized controlled trial. J Am Coll Surg 2001;192:172–9.

[4] Spechler SJ, Lee E, Ahnene D, et al. Long-term outcome of medical and surgical therapies for gastroesophageal reflux disease: follow-up of a randomized controlled trial. JAMA 2001; 285:2331–8.

[5] Liu JY, Woloshin S, Laycock WS, et al. Late outcomes after laprascopic surgery for gastroesophageal reflux. Arch Surg 2002;137:397–401.

[6] Klaus A, Hinder RA, DeVault KR, et al. Bowel dysfunction after laprascopic antireflux surgery: incidence, severity and clinical course. Am J Med 2003;114:6–9.

[7] Huedebert G, Marks L, Wilcox C, et al. Choice of long-term strategy for the manage-ment of patients with severe esophagitis. A cost-utility analysis. Gastroenterology 1997; 112:1078–86.

[8] Swain CP, Mills TN. An endoscopic sewing machine. Gastrointest Endosc 1986;32:36–7.

[9] Kadirkamanathan SS, Evans DF, Gong F, et al. Antireflux operations at flexible endoscopy using endoluminal stiching techniques: an experimental study. Gastrointest Endosc 1996;44: 133–43.

[10] Kadirkamanathan SS, Yasaki E, Evan DF, et al. An ambulant porcine model of acid reflux used to evaluate endoscopic gastroplasty. Gut 1999;44:782–8.

[11] Filipi CJ, Lehman GA, Rothstein RI, et al. Transoral, flexivle endoscopic sutureing for treatment of GERD: a multicenter trial. Gastrointest Endosc 2001;53:416–22.

[12] Rothstein RI, Pohl H, Grove M, et al. Endoscopic gastric placation for the treatment of GERD: two year follow-up results [abstract]. Am J Gastroenterol 2001; 96S:107.

[13] Chen YK, Raijman I, Ben-Menachem, et al. Long-term experience with endoluminal gastroplication (ELGP): clinical and economic outcomes of the US multicenter trial. Gastrointest Endosc 2003;57:AB100.

[14] Rothstein RI, Hynes ML, Groce MR, et al. Endoscopic gastric plication (EndoCinch) for GERD: a randomized, sham-controlled, blinded, single center study. Gastrointest Endosc 2004;59:AB111.

[15] Mahmood Z, Byrne PJ, McCullough J, et al. A comparison of BARD EndoCinch transesophageal endoscopic placation (BETEP) with laproscopic Nissen fundoplication (LNF) for the treatment of gastroesophageal reflux disease (GORD). Gastrointest Endosc 2002;55:AB90.

[16] Chuttani R, Kozarek R, Critchlow J, et al. A novel endoscopic full-thickness plicator for treatment of GERD: an animal model study. Gastrointest Endosc 2002;56:116–22.

[17] Chuttani R, Sud R, Sachdev G, et al. Endoscopic full-thickness plication for GERD: final results on human pilot study. Gastrointest Endosc 2002;55:A258.

[18] Pleskow D, Rothstein RI, Lo S, et al. Endoscopic full-thickness plication for the treatment of GERD: a multicenter tiral. Gastrointest Endosc 2004;59:163–71.

[19] Kim MS, Dent J, Holloway R, et al. Radiofrequency energy delivery to the gastric cardia inhibits triggering of transient lower esophageal sphinter relaxation in a canine model. Gastroenterology 2000;188:AB4790.

[20] Tam WCE, Schoeman MN, Zhang Q, et al. Delivery of radiofrequency energy to the lower oesophageal sphincter and gastric cardia inhibits transient lower oesphageal sphincter relaxations and gastro-oesophageal reflux in patients with reflux disease. Gut 2003;52: 479–85.

[21] Utley DS, Kim MS, Vierra MA, et al. Augmentation of lower esophageal sphincter pressure and gastric yield pressure after radiofrequency delivery to the gastroesophageal junction: a porcine model. Gastrointest Endosc 2000;52:81–6.

[22] Chang K, Utley DS. Endoscopic ultrasound (EUS) in-vivo assessment of radiofrequency (RF) energy delivery to the gastroesophageal (GE) junction in a porcine model. Gastrointest Endosc 2001;53:AB4191.

[23] Triadafilopoulos G, DiBaise JK, Nostrant TT, et al. Radiofrequency energy delivery to the gastroesophageal junction for the treatment of gastroesophageal reflux disease. Gastrointest Endosc 2001;53:407–15.

[24] Triadafilopoulos G, DiBaise JK, Nostrant TT, et al. The Stretta procedure for the treatment of GERD: 6 and 12 month follow-up of the US open label trial. Gastrointest Endosc 2002;55: 149–56.

[25] Triadafilopoulos F. Changes in GERD symptom scores correlate with improvement in esophageal acid exposure after the Stretta procedure. Surg Endosc 2004;18: 1038–44.

[26] Wolfsen HC, Richards WO. The Stretta procedure for the treatment of GERD: a registry of 558 patients. J Laparoendosc Adv Surg Tech A 2002;12:395–402.

[27] Corley DA, Katz P, Wo JM, et al. Improvement of gastroesophageal reflux symptoms after radiofrequency energy: a randomized, sham-controlled trial. Gastroenterology 2003;125: 668–76.

[28] O'Connor KW, Madison SA, Smith DJ, et al. An experimental endoscopic technique for reversing gastroesophageal reflux in dogs by injecting inert material in the distal esophagus. Gastrointest Endosc 1984;30:275–80.

[29] O'Connor KW, Lehman GA. Endoscopic placement of collagen at the lower esophageal sphincter to inhibit gastroesophageal reflux: a pilot study of 10 medically intractable patients. Gastrointest Endosc 1988;34:106–12.

[30] Feretis C, Benakis P, Dimopoulos C, et al. Endoscopic implantation of Plexiglas (PMMA) microspheres for the treatment of GERD. Gastrointest Endosc 2001;53:423–6.

[31] Mason RJ, Hughes M, Lehman GA, et al. Endoscopic augmentation of the cardia with a biocompatible injectable polymer (Enteryx) in a porcine model. Surg Endosc 2002;16:386–91.

[32] Deviere J, Pastorelli A, Louis H, et al. Endoscopic implantation of a biopolymer in the lower esophageal sphincter for gastroesophageal reflux: a pilot study. Gastrointest Endsoc 2002;55:335–41.

[33] Johnson DA, Ganz R, Aisenberg J, et al. Endoscopic, deep mural implantation of Enteryx for the treatment of GERD: 6-month follow-up of a multicenter trial. Am J Gastroenterol 2003;98:250–8.

[34] Johnson DA, Ganz R, Aisenberg J, et al. Endoscopic implantation of Enteryx for treatment of GERD: 12-month results of a prospective, multicenter trial. Am J Gastroenterol 2003;98:1921–30.

[35] Easter DW, Yurek M, Johnson G. Long-term retention of endoscopically placed hydrogel prostheses at the lower esophageal sphincter in pigs. Surg Endosc 2004;18:448–51.

[36] Fockens P, Bruno MJ, Hirsch DP, et al. Endoscopic augmentation of the lower esophageal sphincter. Pilot study of the Gatekeeper Reflux Repair System in patients with GERD. Gastrointest Endosc 2002;55:AB257.

[37] Fockens P, Bruno MJ, Gabbrielli A, et al. Endoscopic augmentation of the lower esophageal sphincter for the treatment of gastroesophageal reflux disease: multicenter study of the Gatekeeper Reflux Repair System. Endoscopy 2004;36:682–9.

splanchnic nerves (sympathetic). The smooth muscle of the stomach consists of an inner circular muscle layer, which is thickest in the area of the antrum, and an outer longitudinal muscle layer. An inner oblique muscle layer is also present in the region of the gastric body-antrum. The pylorus separates the stomach from the duodenal bulb, and consists of a thick band of circular smooth muscle that is approximately 1.5 cm in length. These muscle fibers interdigitate with slips of longitudinal muscle from the antrum; in addition, the pylorus receives support from connective tissue of the mucosal layer and the inner circular muscle layer of the stomach. Anatomically, the pylorus is often thought of as little more than a passive barrier to prevent the too-rapid passage of food from the stomach to the small intestine.

In regard to functional anatomy, however, the stomach is very different from the classical model described above. The stomach is divided into two major functional areas—the "proximal stomach" and the "distal stomach." The proximal stomach consists of the fundus and the upper body. The primary function of the proximal stomach is to accommodate ingested food (see below). The distal stomach consists of the lower body and antrum. This area plays a critical role in the processes of trituration and emptying (see below). In regard to gastric motility and function, the intrinsic nervous system of the stomach is more important than the extrinsic innervation described above. This is because the denervated stomach retains its ability to mix and grind food and empty it into the small intestine. The intrinsic nervous system has three major components: the interstitial cells of Cajal (ICC), the extensive network of fibers that connect the ICC to other nerve cells and ganglia throughout the stomach, and the enteric nervous system (ENS). The ENS is responsible for relaying sensory information from the stomach to the brain via the vagus nerve. The ENS is also responsible for the propagation of motor impulses throughout the stomach. The collection of nerve cells located beneath the mucosa (the submucosal plexus) is predominantly concerned with sensory function; the collection of nerve cells located between the two muscle layers (the myenteric plexus) plays a critical role in gastric motor function. Finally, as described below, the pylorus plays a very active and critical role in both normal and abnormal gastric emptying.

Normal gastric function

Accommodation

Accommodation is the automatic process that occurs in response to eating or drinking. As swallowing is initiated and food enters the stomach, the gastric fundus reflexively relaxes to accommodate the ingested food and liquid. This process occurs via a vaso-vagal reflex. Nitric oxide (NO) and vasoactive intestinal polypeptide (VIP) are two of the neurotransmitters involved in mediating fundic relaxation [1]. Fundic relaxation allows large volumes of food to be stored and accommodated without a concomitant increase in gastric pressure. After food is ingested, it remains in the fundus for a variable amount of time, usually 40 to 60 minutes. The length of time that food remains in the fundus depends upon the volume of the meal, the percentage of liquids versus solids, the caloric content of the material, and the relative contribution of fats, protein, and carbohydrates. This delay in transferring food from the fundus to the body contributes to the initial delay seen in gastric emptying scans (referred to as the lag phase). In contrast to the lower stomach (described below), the fundus has little phasic activity (phasic activity refers to contractile activity of the smooth muscle); rather, the fundus has elevated tone (this refers to resting pressure of the smooth muscle fibers). Food gradually moves from the upper stomach to the lower stomach as a result of the pressure gradient between the fundus (high tone) to the antrum (low tone). After vagotomy, the fundus does not accommodate normally in response to the ingestion of foods [2]. Research studies using a gastric barostat have found that some patients who have non-ulcer dyspepsia also have inadequate fundic relaxation after eating a meal. This may account for complaints of postprandial pain and fullness in patients who have undergone a truncal vagotomy or who have non-ulcer dyspepsia.

Trituration

Trituration is the process of mixing and grinding food in the lower stomach. Recurrent and gentle peristaltic waves mix the food with secreted acid and pepsin, and move the food toward the pylorus. Strong phasic contractions (often over 100 mm Hg) rapidly propel pieces of food toward the closed pylorus. As the food is pushed against the closed pylorus, it breaks into smaller pieces, after which it is retropulsed into the lower stomach so that further mixing can take place [3]. This process may last up to several hours, depending upon the size of the meal, the caloric content, the amount of liquid ingested, and the relative amounts of fat, fiber, protein, and carbohydrates.

Emptying

After the food is properly broken down and mixed, and the caloric content and viscosity are appropriate, small aliquots (3–5 cc) of nearly liquefied food are emptied into the duodenum by gastric peristaltic contractions. This typically occurs when food particles are less than 1 mm in diameter. In general, liquids always empty faster than meals with solid foods, and non-fat meals empty faster than meals high in fat content. Overall, normal gastric emptying is the culmination of a series of complex myoelectrical and mechanical (contractile) events that are influenced by extrinsic (central nervous system) and intrinsic neural activity. In addition, both humoral and hormonal factors, as well as feedback from the small intestine all play critical roles in modulating gastric emptying. Physiologic delays in gastric emptying can occur because of exaggerated fundic relaxation, diminished antral contractions, or heightened pyloroduodenal resistance. Truncal vagotomy decreases gastric emptying of solids, but accelerates emptying of liquids [4].

Antropyloric coordination

The pylorus plays a critical role in the timing of gastric emptying. During trituration, the pyloric sphincter is closed, which results in retropulsion of larger food particles back into the stomach for further mixing. Normal gastric emptying requires that antropyloric coordination be intact; this ensures that antral peristaltic waves are appropriately coordinated with an open pylorus. In addition, duodenal bulb pressures should be low to maximize antral emptying. Pyloric dysfunction may result in either delayed gastric emptying (diabetic gastroparesis, pyloric stenosis [5]) or rapid gastric emptying (due to previous pyloric myotomy or vagotomy).

Evaluating gastric function

There are a number of different methods to assess gastric function and gastric motility. These vary significantly with regard to cost, availability, safety, and level of invasiveness. The most common methods are briefly described below.

Upper gastrointestinal series

The upper gastrointestinal (UGI) series is widely available, inexpensive, and is best used to define anatomy and to rule out a mechanical obstruction. This test is not a measure of gastric function or motility, although prolonged retention of barium in the stomach (>6 hours) is suggestive of gastroparesis.

Upper endoscopy

This test is safe and readily available, although more expensive than a UGI series. It is ideal to assess anatomy, take biopsies, and to rule out a mechanical obstruction. It is not a valid test to measure gastric motility; however, if retained food is found in the stomach after an overnight fast and mechanical obstruction is not present, then gastroparesis is the most likely etiology.

Solid phase gastric emptying scan

This test uses an externally positioned gamma scintillation camera to measure emptying of 99m-Technitium sulfur colloid from the stomach. The sulfur colloid is usually added to scrambled eggs. Advantages to this test include safety, availability, a modest cost, and the noninvasive nature of the test. In addition, gastric emptying scans are considered the best currently available test to evaluate and quantitate gastric emptying. Measurement of gastric emptying should be performed for at least 2 hours, and ideally for 4 hours [6]. The initial lag phase of the test (45–60 minutes) reflects the physiological processes of accommodation and trituration. Gastric emptying of solids then occurs in a linear manner. Unfortunately, gastric emptying scans are still not standardized among hospitals, and therefore it is very difficult to compare data from different institutions. In addition, there is poor correlation between patients' symptoms and the results of gastric emptying scans. Liquid gastric emptying scans are of little value and should not be routinely performed.

Electrogastrography

Electrogastrography (EGG) measures electrical activity in the stomach and in many ways is similar to an electrocardiogram. First, the skin is gently abraded before placement of the electrodes. Next, three to four electrodes are positioned in the epigastric area [7]. Baseline recordings are taken for 45 to 60 minutes in the fasting period, and the patient then ingests a standard liquid meal (which differs between different institutions). Postprandial recordings are obtained for another 45 to 60 minutes, and the patient is then discharged to home. This test is very safe and is relatively easy to perform; however, EGG is currently only available at specialized centers because of the cost of the equipment and the need for staff who have specialized training in reading and interpreting the data and tracings.

Antroduodenal manometry

A specially constructed catheter is inserted through the nose and then passed into the stomach and small intestine. Pressure transducers record contractions in the stomach and small intestine. Catheters can be placed either at the time of upper endoscopy, or during fluoroscopy. Proper placement is verified with an abdominal radiograph. This test can be used to differentiate gastric motility problems from small-bowel motility problems, and can also assess whether the underlying problem is a neuropathic process or a myopathic process. In addition, the patient can be tested in both fasting and fed conditions, and medication challenges (ie, erythromycin, octreotide) can be provided. This test is only available at specialized centers because the equipment is expensive and interpretation of the tracings requires specialized training [6].

Other tests

Ultrasound of the stomach, radio-labeled breath tests, positron emission tomography (PET) scans, and MRIs have all been tested in the research setting as alternatives to the tests described above. At present, these tests are all considered experimental. Some patients who have persistent symptoms may require diagnostic laparotomy to biopsy the stomach or small intestine and determine if an infiltrative process (ie, amyloid lymphoma) is present.

Normal gastric motility: electromechanical activity

Pacemaker region/activity

The pacesetter potential arises from an ill-defined collection of cells on the greater curvature of the stomach. These cells, the ICC, are located between the outer longitudinal and the inner circular muscle layers [8]. Unlike the heart, the stomach does not have specialized pathways to conduct these electrical signals. Rather, the pacesetter potential migrates circumferentially and distally from the corpus toward the pylorus, directly through the muscle layers, at a rate of three cycles per minute (cpm) [9]. The pacesetter potential, also called the gastric slow wave, does not migrate into the fundus—this area is "electrically silent" to a large degree. The gastric slow wave is not of significant strength or amplitude to induce a contraction of gastric smooth muscle. Rather, the pacesetter potential sets the frequency of gastric contractions, and this frequency can be modulated by vagal, splanchnic, and hormonal input. If appropriate stimulation is present (either neural or humoral), then the duration and the amplitude of the gastric slow wave is increased, the cell can depolarize, and a phasic contraction occurs (Fig. 1). Thus, the maximum frequency with which the antrum can contract is 3 cpm, although the strength of the contraction can be greatly influenced by both neural and hormonal factors. After vagotomy, the pacemaker becomes disorganized and the electrical rhythm is disturbed; however, after several months new pacemakers may take over—these are typically located in the antrum.

Normal gastric myoelectrical activity

The smooth muscle of the gut is characterized by tone (sustained tension), upon which phasic contractions are superimposed. The upper stomach has high tone, but little or no phasic activity. In contrast, the antrum has very low tone but significant phasic (contractile) activity. As noted above, contractile activity in the antrum depends upon both the underlying slow gastric rhythm and a variety of modulating factors that determine the timing and strength of phasic contractions.

Gastric motility is generally divided into two basic motor patterns— fasting and fed [10]. The fasting pattern consists of cyclic repetitions between a quiescent state, called Phase I, and periods of contractile activity, labeled Phase II or Phase III of the migrating motor complex (MMC). These three phases of the MMC are seen during fasting, are inhibited by eating, and generally occur every 90 to 120 minutes (Fig. 2). The most characteristic of

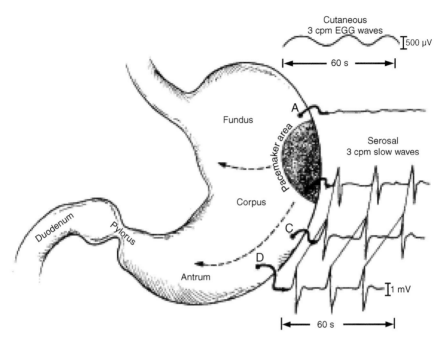

Fig. 1. ICC and pacer and waves of contraction. Gastric slow waves or pacesetter potentials are rhythmic depolarization and repolarization waves that begin in the pacemaker region. Slow waves migrate circumferentially as indicated by the horizontal arrow and, at the same time, migrate distally as shown by the arrow pointing to the antrum. In this figure, there are three electrodes on the gastric body and antrum and one electrode on the fundus. Note that a slow-wave sequence migrates from the pacemaker area into the antrum approximately every 20 seconds or 3 cpm. The recording from the fundus, however, indicates no electrical rhythmicity. Also shown are cutaneous 3 cpm EGG waves. The 3 cpm EGG waves represent the summation of electrical events from the stomach as measured from the cutaneous or surface electrodes. The surface recording of the stomach myoelectrical activity is an EGG. (*From* Koch KL. The stomach. In: Schuster MM, editor. Atlas of gastrointestinal motility in health and disease. Baltimore [MD]: Williams and Wilkins; 1993. p. 165; with permission.)

these patterns is Phase III, which begins in the antrum. Phase III consists of strong, regular, rhythmic contractions that typically occur at a frequency of 3 cpm and can approach 100 to 150 mm Hg in amplitude. Phase III typically last 5 to 10 minutes. The function of Phase III is to clear the indigestible fibrous material from the stomach and to move such debris through the small intestine and into the colon. Phase I always follows Phase III of the MMC and is a period of quiescence. Phase I usually lasts 45 to 60 minutes. Irregular, single contractions typify Phase II of the MMC; this phase usually lasts 45 to 50 minutes.

The fed pattern develops 5 to 10 minutes after eating, and consists of irregular but persistent contractile activity that is designed to mix and grind food, and then propel it toward the antrum. This pattern interrupts the fasting pattern wherever it is in the cycle (Fig. 3). The length of the fed

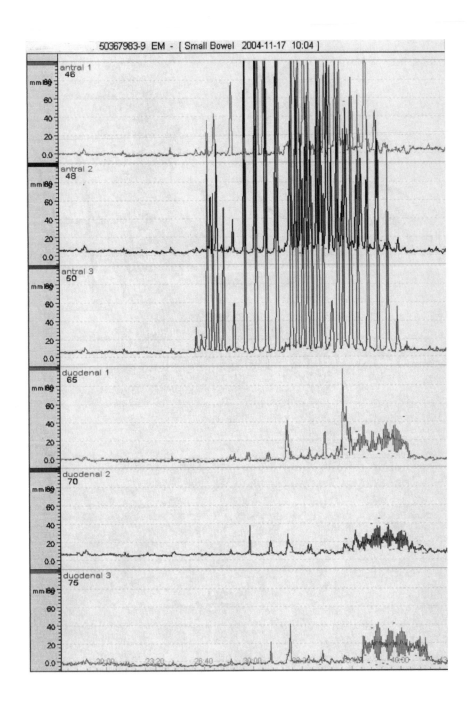

pattern depends upon the size and content of the meal; typically it lasts for several hours.

Gastroparesis

Definition

Gastroparesis is defined as the impaired transit of intraluminal contents from the stomach to the duodenum in the absence of mechanical obstruction. Symptoms cannot help discriminate between mechanical causes of gastric outlet obstruction versus true gastroparesis, and thus mechanical reasons (peptic ulcer, tumor) need to be ruled out first. This can be done with either an esophagogastroduodenoscopy (EGD) or UGI series.

Etiology

There are multiple etiologies of gastroparesis and these are listed in Box 1. The most common reason for gastroparesis to occur is still not known, because idiopathic gastroparesis accounts for approximately 50% of all cases. A majority of these cases may be postviral in nature. Diabetes accounts for 25% of cases, and this is most likely to occur in patients who have long-standing Type I diabetes and associated neuropathy, nephropathy, and retinopathy [11]. Other causes for gastroparesis include collagen-vascular disorders (5%), intestinal pseudo-obstruction (5%), and prior surgery involving the stomach (10%). Although the prevalence of gastroparesis from prior ulcer surgery has significantly decreased due to the efficacy of proton pump inhibitors (PPIs), the number of cases of gastroparesis developing after antireflux surgery is increasing. This likely reflects vagal nerve injury at the time of fundoplication.

Pathophysiology

A number of different physiologic processes have been implicated in the genesis of gastroparesis. These are briefly noted below:

1. Impaired fundal tone. Low tone prevents or delays the normal movement of gastric contents from the fundus into the antrum.

Fig. 2. Antroduodenal manometry showing normal fasting MMC. Phase I of the MMC is noted in the antrum in the first part of the tracing. The antrum is quiescent during Phase I of the MMC (far left hand side of the panel). Irregular, single contractions typify Phase II of the MMC. This period typically lasts 40–50 minutes, and culminates in the regular Phase III contractions of the MMC, which last 5–10 minutes (far right side of panel). Normal antral activity usually occurs at a frequency of 3 cpm. Phase III contractions originate in the antrum approximately 70% of the time, and they migrate through the duodenum and small intestine. Approximately 30% of the time, Phase III contractions originate in the duodenum and migrate distally to the ileum. The small intestine has a different pattern of motility, characterized by a faster frequency (9–12 cpm) and lower-amplitude contractions.

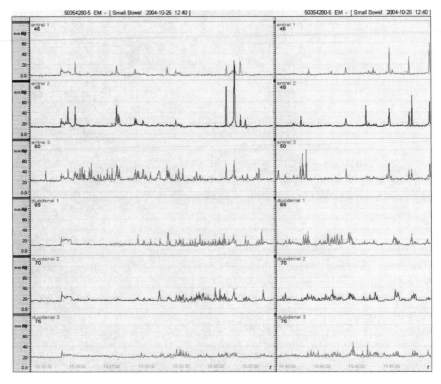

Fig. 3. Antroduodenal manometry showing normal fed MMC. Sporadic irregular contractions are seen in the stomach before eating a meal. The patient is then given a standard liquid meal that is ingested over 5–10 minutes. After ingesting a meal, high-amplitude but irregular contractions are seen in the antrum, while irregular but lower-amplitude contractions are seen in the small intestine.

2. Antral hypomotility. A weak "antral pump" prolongs trituration and delays the passage of food from the stomach into the duodenum.

3. Antroduodenal dyscoordination. Poor coordination between the antrum and duodenum, or spasm of the pylorus (pylorospasm), prevents normal passage of material from the stomach into the small intestine.

4. Gastric pacemaker dysrhythmias. This includes bradygastria (the pacemaker is too slow), tachygastria (the pacemaker is too fast), and other arrhythmias. Bradygastria can lead to infrequent antral contractions, whereas tachygastria can lead to inefficient coupling of the electrical signal to smooth muscle cells.

5. Excessive inhibitory feedback from the small bowel to the stomach can delay gastric emptying. Mediators involved in this may include cholecystokinin (CCK) and somatostatin.

Symptoms

The most common symptoms of gastroparesis are nausea, vomiting, early satiety, anorexia, and weight loss. Epigastric pain is an often overlooked symptom of gastroparesis, although it may occur in up to 80% of patients [12]. Although less common, some patients only have persistent complaints of bloating or difficult to control reflux symptoms. Postprandial fullness and vomiting are two symptoms that are most likely to predict the presence of gastroparesis [13].

Physical examination

Most patients who have gastroparesis have some abdominal distention and tympany. Tenderness may be present in the epigastric area, and a succussion splash may occasionally be heard. Abdominal bruits should be listened for, and a thorough examination should be performed to rule out masses, ascites, and lymphadenopathy. Blood pressure, pulse, skin turgor, axillary sweat, and mucous membranes should all be assessed to look for evidence of dehydration. A malar rash may be seen in patients who have systemic lupus erythematosus (SLE), and sclerodactyly and calcinosis should be sought out in those patients who have possible scleroderma.

Laboratory tests

These are generally normal in most patients who have gastroparesis. Severe vomiting may produce hypokalemia and a contraction alkalosis. A complete blood count, serum electrolytes, and a serum albumin should be ordered on the first visit. Special blood work may be required to help identify the underlying cause of gastroparesis, such as an autoimmune disorder, a metabolic disorder, or a paraneoplastic syndrome. Laboratory studies that may need to be ordered in these cases include: HgbA1c, thyroid function tests, erythrocyte sedimentation rate, calcium, para-thyroid hormone, cortisol, serum protein electrophoresis, anti-nuclear antibody, anti-mitochondrial antibody, anti-smooth muscle antibody, anti-Hu antibody, and Lyme titer.

Differential diagnosis

Because nearly all of the symptoms of gastroparesis are quite nonspecific, there is a long list of disorders that need to be considered during the evaluation process. These other conditions include dyspepsia, peptic ulcer disease, gastroesophageal reflux disease, gastritis, choledocholithiasis, mesenteric ischemia, pancreatitis, sphincter of Oddi dysfunction, gastric cancer, rumination syndrome, cyclic vomiting syndrome, and psychiatric disorders (anorexia, bulimia). If symptoms are associated with disordered

Box 1. Etiologies of gastroparesis

Neuromuscular
Diabetes
Amyloid
Parkinson's
Shy Drager syndrome
Muscular (myotonic dystrophy)
Scleroderma and other connective tissue diseases (CTDs)
Hollow visceral neuropathy or myopathy
Duchenne's muscular dystrophy

Infiltrative
Malignancy
Amyloid

Infectious
Postviral (chronic)
Herpes zoster
Lyme disease
Trypanosoma cruzi
Acute viral (Norwalk)
Clostridium botulinum
Epstein-Barr virus

Postsurgical
Vagotomy (truncal or selective)
Partial or total gastrectomy
Scarring/adhesions

Psychiatric
Anorexia
Bulimia

Metabolic
Hyperglycemia
Renal insufficiency
Hypo- or hyperthyroidism
Hypo- or hyperparathyroidism

Idiopathic
Bradygastria
Tachygastria
Other pacemaker arrythmias

Medications
May cause gastroparesis
  Anticholinergics
  Opiates
  L-dopa
  Tricyclic antidepressants
  Phenothiazines
  Somatostatin (high dose)
Rarely cause gastroparesis
  Calcium channel blockers
  Sympathomimetics
  Progesterone
  Cannabis
  Aluminum antacids
  Gamma-aminobutyric acid
  Cholera toxin
  Nicotine
  Alcohol
  Sucralfate

Other
Ischemia
Radiation
Chronic intestinal pseudo-obstruction (CIP)
Cirrhosis
Median arcuate ligament syndrome
Paraneoplastic syndrome
Prior organ transplant
Pancreatitis

defecation, then irritable bowel syndrome (IBS) is the likely diagnosis. Dyspepsia is one of the most common diagnoses confused with gastroparesis. Dyspepsia is more prevalent than gastroparesis, although it is rarely associated with significant nausea and vomiting. A large number of patients who have dyspepsia have symptoms of early satiety and postprandial nausea, however, and 30% to 50% of patients who have dyspepsia may have a mild delay in gastric emptying [13].

Complications

The most common complications seen in patients who have gastroparesis are weight loss, malnutrition, electrolyte disorders, Mallory-Weiss tear from repeated vomiting, bezoar formation, aspiration pneumonia, and unnecessary surgery (ie, cholecystectomy).

Treatment

The goals of treatment include relief of symptoms, improved nutrition, better glycemic control in diabetics, and prevention of complications (ie, bezoar formation). In some cases, medications can be used only when the patient is symptomatic, although in most cases chronic therapy is required. Therapeutic considerations of drug therapy should include: the need to treat both nausea and vomiting, an appropriate dosing schedule and route of administration (oral, subcuteneous, intravenous), drug availability, medication costs, and the risk/benefit ratio of the drugs. A therapeutic trial should be at least 4 to 8 weeks in length, because many patients do not realize any benefit during the first 1 to 3 weeks of therapy. In addition, because therapeutic options are limited, it is important to give each medication a fair trial before deciding that the medication has not been effective.

Diet

Small, frequent meals are a mainstay of therapy. They should be low in fiber (to prevent bezoar formation), and low in fat (fat delays gastric emptying). Liquids should be emphasized over solid foods. Strict control of serum glucose is critical in diabetics, because hyperglycemia further delays gastric emptying [14].

Exercise

Postprandial exercise (walking, biking) has been shown to increase the normal 3 cpm activity in the stomach, and thus may improve gastric emptying in some patients [15].

Medications

Metoclopramide. Metoclopramide is a substituted benzamide [16]. It acts as a cholinomimetic to release acetylcholine (Ach) from intrinsic neurons in the gut. It also blocks dopamine receptors, which leads to inhibition of receptive relaxation in the fundus and thus improves the transfer of food from the fundus to the antrum. Metoclopramide increases the tone and amplitude of antral contractions, and thus increases peristalsis. Metoclopramide also relaxes the pylorus to a small degree, which further aids gastric emptying. Anti-emetic effects are due to blockade of dopamine (DA) receptors in the chemoreceptor trigger zone of the fourth ventricle. Metoclopramide can be given orally, subcutaneously, or intravenously. For oral doses, the authors recommend starting at a low dose of 10 mg twice daily, and then slowly increasing to 20 mg orally four times a day over the course of 1 to 2 months, while carefully watching for side effects or adverse events. Unfortunately, side effects develop in 20% to 40% of patients. These may include mild sedation or agitation, but may also involve extrapyramidal side effects such as tremor, akathisia, and tardive dyskinesia. Tardive dyskinesia is more likely to occur in diabetics than nondiabetics. Other side effects include gynecomastia, galactorrhea, mastalgia, impotence, and menstrual irregularities.

Erythromycin. Erythromycin is a very potent gastrokinetic. It is a macrolide antibiotic that acts as a motilin agonist [17]. Erythromycin induces Phase III of the MMC, and also increases the number and amplitude of antral contractions. It is best given in liquid form (erythromycin oral suspension), using 50 to 100 mg orally four times a day, given 30 to 45 minutes before each of the three main meals and at bedtime. Higher doses are not more effective, and often cause nausea or abdominal discomfort. Patients usually note improvement in symptoms of early satiety, fullness, and vomiting, although erythromycin does not improve symptoms of nausea. Unfortunately, for those patients who respond to this medication, most develop tachyphylaxis after several weeks of therapy. If the patient is given a drug-free holiday of 4 to 6 weeks, and the medication is restarted, most patients again note an improvement in their symptoms. Side effects include nausea, vomiting, abdominal cramps or discomfort, and occasionally, diarrhea.

Domperidone. This is a benzamidazole derivative. To some degree, domperidone acts like metoclopramide. It is both a prokinetic and an anti-emetic, and works by blocking dopamine receptors [18]. Unlike metoclopramide, however, it does not cross the blood-brain barrier, and thus does not cause sedation, agitation, or tardive dyskinesia. Side effects occur in up to 7% to 10% of patients treated with domperidone, and include mastalgia, gynecomastia, galactorrhea, impotence, and menstrual irregularities. Domperidone is only available in oral form. The authors generally recommend starting patients at 10 mg twice a day, and then slowly advancing to 20 mg orally four times a day over the course of 4 to 8 weeks, while carefully monitoring the patient for side effects. Unfortunately, this drug is not available in the United States; however, patients can obtain it from Canada, New Zealand, and many other countries in Europe and Latin America.

Tegaserod. Tegaserod is a selective 5-HT4 agonist approved by the Food and Drug Administration (FDA) for treatment of chronic constipation in men and women, and IBS and constipation in women. Research studies have shown that it increases gastric emptying in diabetic mice, increases gastric emptying in patients who have dyspepsia and delayed gastric emptying, and increases orocecal transit time in women who have constipation [19,20]. Tegaserod does not cross the blood-brain barrier, and thus does not have the central nervous system (CNS) side effects commonly noted with metoclopramide. Tegaserod is not yet approved by the FDA for use in gastroparetic patients.

Anti-emetics. There are a large number of anti-emetics that can be used to treat nausea in patients who have gastroparesis. A complete review of all anti-emetic agents is beyond the scope of this article; however, many patients who have severe symptoms require more than one anti-emetic at a time. In these patients, the authors recommend that one agent from each of several different categories be used, rather than two agents from the same general category (eg, a phenothiazine, plus a 5-HT3 antagonist such as ondansetron). A selection of anti-emetics is provided in Box 2.

Box 2. Medications commonly used to treat nausea

Antihistamines
Dimenhydrinate
Meclizine
Diphenhydramine

Anticholinergic agents
Scopolamine
Hyoscine

Phenothiazines
Prochlorperazine
Promethazine
Chlorpromazine

Butyrophenones
Haloperidol
Droperidol

Dopaminergic antagonists
Metoclopramide
Domperidone

5-HT3 antagonists
Ondansetron
Granisetron
Dolasetron

Miscellaneous
Ginger
Lorazempam
Dronabinol
Prednisone

Botulinum toxin injection of the pylorus. Botulinum toxin inhibits the release of acetylcholine from synaptic vesicles at the synaptic junction, thereby inducing a state of transient muscle paralysis [21]. The authors' laboratory has shown that botulinum toxin injection of the pylorus decreases pyloric resting tone and pylorospasm, relieves symptoms of nausea and vomiting, and improves gastric emptying in patients who have diabetic gastroparesis [22]. Similar work by Miller and colleagues [23] showed that botulinum toxin injection of the pylorus improved symptoms in patients who have idiopathic gastroparesis. At present, this treatment is mostly performed in the research setting or in clinical trials. Further work is necessary to assess long-term outcomes.

Gastric stimulation. See the following section.

Total parenteral nutrition. For those patients who have persistent symptoms of nausea and vomiting with nutritional compromise, total parenteral nutrition (TPN) is sometimes required. The potential complications of blood clots and infections are well-known.

Jejunal-tube feedings. For patients who are unable to take in enough calories to maintain normal nutrition, a jejunal (J)-tube is often beneficial. This can be placed endoscopically, surgically, or by interventional radiology. We do not recommend G-tube placement for patients who have gastroparesis, because the formula is infused into an organ that does not empty properly.

Gastric pacing and gastric stimulation

Multiple pathophysiologic abnormalities can lead to the clinical presentation of gastroparesis. Disordered gastric myoelectrical is a common finding in patients who have gastroparesis. In a small case-control study by Bortolotti and colleagues [24], normal volunteers were found to have pacesetter potentials at a regular frequency of approximately three per minute, associated with the generation of pressure waves. In contrast, patients who have chronic idiopathic gastroparesis were found to have a variety of electrical dysrhythmias, ranging from premature spike potentials to brady- or tachyarrhythmias. Myoelectric activity correlated with these manometric findings, suggesting that antral hypomotility may be related to the absence of regular occurrence of pacesetter potentials.

Identification of the relationship between gastric myoelectric activity and gastric hypomotility prompted researchers to investigate the effects of electrical stimulation on gastric motility [25]. There are currently two major techniques for electrically stimulating the stomach: (1) high-energy, long-duration pulses, and (2) high-frequency, low-energy with short pulses.

Electrical stimulation using high-energy, long-duration pulses occurs at a frequency 10% higher than that of the intrinsic slow wave. The pulses entrain the gastric slow wave and change the underlying rhythm of the stomach, as demonstrated in small case series of patients who have gastroparetic symptoms [25]. Entraining and accelerating the gastric slow wave may also improve gastric emptying. In a second case series of nine patients who had intractable gastroparesis [26], an external pacing device was placed. This device consisted of four pairs of cardiac pacing wires implanted on the serosa of the stomach, brought out through the abdominal wall and connected to a portable, external pacemaker. After 2 to 3 months of gastric pacing, eight of nine patients no longer required J-tube feedings. In this uncontrolled study, mean gastric retention at two hours fell from 77% to 56% ($P < 0.04$).

More recently, gastric electrical stimulation (GES) has been used to treat patients who have either idiopathic or diabetic gastroparesis. This method employs an implantable neurostimulator that delivers a high-frequency, low-energy signal with short pulses. This device uses stimulating leads sutured into the gastric muscle along the greater curvature of the stomach. These leads are then attached to the electric stimulator, which is placed into a subcutaneous pocket on the abdominal wall. Unlike the long duration pulses, this stimulator does not entrain slow waves or change underlying slow-wave dysrhythmias. Preliminary results were encouraging; an initial study showed a decrease in nausea and vomiting in 20 of 26 patients at 3 and 6 months after implantation [27]. In long-term follow-up, however, 3 of these patient required total gastrectomy because of continued intractable symptoms of nausea and vomiting, and 3 required device removal because of erosion or device infection.

A second study using the implantable neurostimulator consisted of a double-blind, sham stimulation-controlled trial for 2 months, followed by activation of all devices for 1 year [28]. The study consisted of 33 patients who had either diabetic or idiopathic gastroparesis. This 12-month study was conducted in two phases. Thirty-three patients enrolled had either diabetic or idiopathic gastroparesis. The first phase was a 2-month, double-blind, placebo-controlled, randomized crossover trial, followed by a 10-month open-label period. In the first month, each patient was randomized to either the ON or OFF mode. At the end of the month, the mode was changed to the opposite one. At this time, while still blinded, each patient was asked for his preference (month 1 or month 2). Twenty-one of 33 preferred having the stimulator in the ON mode. In phase 2 of the trial, all devices were turned on. Follow-up at the end of 1 year showed a relative decrease in vomiting frequency from 25 to 6 times per week, with associated improvements in quality of life, primarily in the diabetic gastroparesis subgroup. Several other small case series support the use of GES in refractory gastroparesis [29–31]. Although frequency and severity of nausea and vomiting seems to improve with GES, one small, single-center case series found that patients who had idiopathic gastroparesis and significant abdominal pain did not respond to GES [32].

Poor nutritional status is common in patients who have refractory gastroparesis. A subset of 12 patients in the Gastric Electromechanical Stimulation (GEMS) Study Group underwent nutritional assessment, including measurement of albumin, weight, and body mass index, before and up to 5 years after implantation of a GES [33]. GES resulted not only in rapid improvement in symptoms, but also resulted in improvement in body weight, body mass index, and serum albumin at 3 to 6 months. At 1, 2, and 5 years, weight gain was maintained.

Based in part of these results, the neurostimulator was granted humanitarian-use device approval from the FDA for the treatment of chronic refractory nausea and vomiting. At present, the primary complication has been localized infection occurring at rates of 5% to 10%, not significantly different from the rates associated with cardiac pacemaker placement. At this time, the greatest limiting factor for device implantation is its cost, especially in the context of only modest improvements in disease-specific quality of life. At one institution, the implantation cost was estimated at $20,000 per patient [34]. Certainly, for GES to become a viable option for medically refractory gastroparesis, researchers will be challenged to demonstrate continued patient improvement with the GES device and to demonstrate that the improvement in the disabling features of gastroparesis results in reduction of hospitalization, health care use, and thereby health care cost.

Summary

The stomach is an amazing organ, with both sensory and motor functions. The stomach is functionally divided into two major areas: the proximal stomach accommodates ingested food via the vaso-vagal reflex, and the distal stomach triturates and empties the ingested food. When this system is disrupted, such as by impaired fundal tone, antral hypomotility, or antroduodenal dyscoordination, normal gastric emptying is compromised and patients may develop gastroparesis.

Symptoms of gastroparesis are common and nonspecific, which explains why gastroparesis is often overlooked in the differential diagnosis of patients who have chronic symptoms of nausea, vomiting, early satiety, anorexia, and weight loss. Because we cannot discriminate between mechanical causes of gastric outlet obstruction and gastroparesis on the basis of symptoms, mechanical reasons (peptic ulcer, tumor) need to be ruled out first. This can be done with either an EGD or UGI series.

A number of tools are now available to assess gastric function and motility, including solid-phase gastric emptying scans, EGG and antroduodenal manometry. UGI series and EGD, though often part of the evaluation of a patient who has suspected gastric motor dysfuntion, do not provide information on function or motility.

Treatment options for patients who have delayed gastric emptying include dietary modifications, exercise, the use of both prokinetic and anti-emetic agents, and botulinum toxin injection of the pylorus. Most recently, surgical intervention for refractory gastroparesis has been explored, using an implantable gastric neurostimulator.

References

[1] Murray J, Du C, Ledlow A, et al. Nitric oxide: mediator of nonadrenergic noncholinergic nerve-induced responses of opossum esophageal muscle. Am J Physiol 1991;261:G401–6.

[2] Jahnberg T, Abrahamsson H, Jansson G, et al. Gastric relaxatory response to feeding before and after vagotomy. Scand J Gastroenterol 1977;12:225–8.

[3] Houghton LA, Read NW, Heddle R, et al. Relationship of the motor activity of the antrum, pylorus, and duodenum to gastric emptying of a solid-liquid mixed meal. Gastroenterology 1988;94:1285–91.

[4] Sheiner HJ, Quinlan MF, Thompson IJ. Gastric motility and emptying in normal and post-vagotomy subjects. Gut 1980;21:753–9.

[5] Mearin F, Camilleri M, Malagelada JR. Pyloric dysfunction in diabetics with recurrent nausea and vomiting. Gastroenterology 1986;90:1919–25.

[6] Camilleri M, Hasler W, Parkman HP, et al. Measurement of gastroduodenal motility in the GI laboratory. Gastroenterology 1998;115:747–62.

[7] Koch KL, Stern RM, editors. Handbook of electrogastrography. New York: Oxford University Press; 2004.

[8] Zarate N, Mearin F, Wang XY, et al. Severe idiopathic gastroparesis due to neuronal and interstitial cells of Cajal degeneration: pathological findings and management. Gut 2003;52: 966–70.

[9] Hinder RA, Kelly KA. Human gastric pacesetter potential: site of origin, spread, and response to gastric transaction and proximal gastric Vagotomy. Am J Surg 1977;133:29–33.

[10] Geldof H, van der Schee EJ, Grashuis JL. Electrogastrographic characteristics of the interdigestive migrating complex in humans. Am J Physiol 1986;250:G165–71.

[11] Soykan I, Sivri B, Sarosiek I, et al. Demography, clinical characteristics, psychological profiles, treatment, and long-term follow-up of patients with gastroparesis. Dig Dis Sci 1998; 43:2398–404.

[12] Hoogerwerf WA, Pasricha PJ, Kalloo AN, et al. Pain: the overlooked symptom in gastroparesis. Am J Gastroenterol 1999;94:1029–33.

[13] Stanghellini V, Tosetti C, Paternico A, et al. Risk indicators of delayed gastric emptying of solids in patients with functional dyspepsia. Gastroenterology 1996;110:1036–42.

[14] Jebbink RJA, Samsom M, Bruijs PPM, et al. Hyperglycemia induces abnormalities of gastric myoelectrical activity in patients with type 1 diabetes mellitus. Gastroenterology 1994;107: 1390–7.

[15] Lu C-L, Shidler N, Chen JDZ. Enhanced postprandial gastric myoelectrical activity after moderate-intensity exercise. Am J Gastroenterol 2000;95:425–31.

[16] Albibi R, McCallum RW. Metoclopramide: pharmacology and clinical application. Ann Intern Med 1983;98:86–95.

[17] Anese V, Janssens J, Vantrappen G, et al. Erythromycin accelerates gastric emptying by inducing antral contractions and improved gastroduodenal coordination. Gastroenterology 1992;102:823–8.

[18] Soykan I, Sarosiek I, McCallum RW. The effect of chronic oral domperidone therapy on gastrointestinal symptoms, gastric emptying, and quality of life in patients with gastroparesis. Am J Gastroenterol 1997;92:976–80.

[19] Lacy BE, Yu S. Tegaserod: a new 5–HT4 agonist. J Clin Gastroenterol 2002;34:27–33.

[20] Tougas G, Chen Y, Luo D, et al. Tegaserod improves gastric emptying in patients with gastroparesis and dyspeptic symptoms. Gastroenterology 2003;124:A468.

[21] Kao I, Drachman DB, Price DL. Botulinum toxin: mechanism of presynaptic blockade. Science 1976;193:1256–8.

[22] Lacy BE, Crowell MD, Schettler-Duncan A, et al. The treatment of diabetic gastroparesis with botulinum toxin injection of the pylorus. Diabetes Care 2004;27:2341–7.

[23] Miller LS, Szych GA, Kantor SB, et al. Treatment of idiopathic gastroparesis with injection of botulinum toxin into the pyloric sphincter muscle. Am J Gastroenterol 2002;97:1653–60.

[24] Bortolotti M, Sarti P, Barbara L, et al. Gastric myoelectric activity in patients with chronic idiopathic gastroparesis. Journal of Gastrointestinal Motility 1990;2(2):104–8.

[25] Parkman HP, Hasler WL, Fisher RS. AGA technical review on the diagnosis and treatment of gastroparesis. Gastroenterol 2004;127:1592–622.

[26] McCallum RW, Chen JZ, Lin Z, et al. Gastric pacing improves emptying and symptoms in patients with gastroparesis. Gastroenterol 1998;114:456–61.

[27] Abell TL, Van Cutsem E, Abrahamsson H, et al. Gastric electrical stimulation in intractable symptomatic gastroparesis. Digestion 2002;66:204–12.

[28] Abell T, McCallum R, Hocking M, et al. Gastric electrical stimulation for medically refractory gastroparesis. Gastroenterol 2003;125:421–8.

[29] Forster J, Sarosiek I, Delcore R, et al. Gastric pacing is a new surgical treatment for gastroparesis. Am J Surg 2001;182:676–81.

[30] McCallum RW, Sarosiek I, Lin Z, et al. Gastric electrical stimulation improves symptoms in patients with drug refractory gastroparesis [abstract]. Am J Gastroenterol 2002;97:S556.

[31] Sobrino M, Patterson DJ, Thirlby RC. Health-related quality of life with gastric stimulation for gastroparesis [abstract]. Am J Gastroenterol 2002;97:S557.

[32] Skole KS, Panganamamula KV, Bromer MQ, et al. Efficacy of gastric electrical stimulation for gastroparesis refractory to medical therapy: a single center experience [abstract]. Am J Gastroenterol 2002;97:S557.

[33] Abell T, Lou J, Tabbaa M, et al. Gastric stimulation for gastroparesis improves nutritional parameters at short, intermediate, and long-term follow-up. JPEN J Parenter Enteral Nutr 2003;27:277–81.

[34] Jones MP, Ebert C, Murayama K: Enterra for gastroparesis [letter]. Am J Gastroenterol 2003;98:2578.

ELSEVIER
SAUNDERS

SURGICAL
CLINICS OF
NORTH AMERICA

Surg Clin N Am 85 (2005) 989–1007

Endoluminal Gastric Surgery: the Modern Era of Minimally Invasive Surgery

Michael J. Rosen, MD[a],
B. Todd Heniford, MD[b],*

[a]Case Western Reserve, Cleveland, OH 44106, USA
[b]Division of Gastrointestinal and Minimal Access Surgery, Carolinas Medical Center,
P.O. Box 32861, Charlotte, NC 28232, USA

Since the advent of the laparoscopic cholecystectomy in 1987, minimally invasive surgery has revolutionized the way we take care of our patients. Laparoscopy has improved patient outcomes across various surgical fields, including thoracic, vascular, and general surgery. With the improvements in laparoscopic skills, the miniaturization of technology, and the fusion of laparoscopy and endoscopy, the next era of surgical growth has begun: endoluminal gastrointestinal surgery. These techniques are a natural extension of conventional laparoscopic surgery. The working space is created within the intestinal lumen, or perhaps the bladder. Using a variety of access devices, we can now operate within the lumen of the organ using laparoscopic instrumentation under endoscopic guidance. The process was initially described in Japan for the local resection of gastric mucosa [1].

The stomach is particularly suited for an endoluminal approach. The distensibility and rather large intraluminal space within the stomach provides adequate working space for laparoscopic instrumentation. When the stomach is fully distended, it approximates the anterior abdominal wall, making percutaneous access safe and effective. It is also reasonably sterile. In addition, the stomach and gastroesophageal (GE) junction contain several types of lesions that require only simple excision. The posterior stomach and GE junctions are also somewhat difficult areas to expose using conventional open techniques, often requiring a potentially morbid upper abdominal incision. Although the standard laparoscopic approach improves

---

* Corresponding author.
   E-mail address: theniford@carolinas.org (B.T. Heniford).

the visualization of the proximal foregut, intraperitoneal fat can impede exposure of the GE junction in obese patients. An endoluminal approach avoids these technical difficulties while maintaining excellent visualization. With these realizations, several pioneering surgeons have begun to define the role of endoluminal gastric surgery.

Endoluminal gastric surgery includes the resection of gastric-based lesions from within the gastric lumen, or use of the stomach as a working space to approach the organ of interest, in pancreatic pseudocyst drainage, for example. This article characterizes the technical approaches to performing endoluminal gastric surgery, the current indications for endoluminal gastric surgery, and the recently reported encouraging data with this novel technique.

Endoluminal transgastric surgical techniques

A summary of the necessary laparoscopic and endoscopic equipment necessary to perform endoluminal intragastric surgery is found in Box 1.

Surgical procedure

After induction of general anesthesia, the endotracheal tube is carefully secured to the lower lip or jaw of the patient. The patient is positioned on the split-leg table with the surgeon in-between the legs and the first assistant on the patient's left (Fig. 1). The flexible endoscopist is stationed at the head of the table. The surgeon should have visual access to both the endoscopic and laparoscopic monitors.

The abdomen is accessed at the umbilicus. A diagnostic laparoscopy is performed to evaluate the peritoneal cavity for evidence of metastatic disease or full-thickness tumor penetration, depending on the indications for the procedure. A laparoscopic ultrasound of the liver can also be performed. The flexible endoscope is then placed transorally, and the pathologic lesion is localized. The locations of the transgastric trocars are determined by the indications for the procedure and the location of the lesion. General principles include obtaining maximal distance in between each trocar (at least 6 cm) while avoiding traversing other intra-abdominal viscera. As the stomach is distended with air, the optimal site of transgastric placement can be localized, under endoscopic guidance, along the greater curvature, by depressing the stomach intraperitoneally. Before placing transgastric trocars, the stomach should be maximally inflated. Typically, the pneumo-peritoneum pressure is decreased to achieve gastric approximation to the abdominal wall. If substantial gastric distension is difficult to achieve with the endoscope, the laparoscopic insufflator is passed through the flexible endoscope via the biopsy channel to provide adequate pressures in order to obtain maximal distension, but this is rarely needed. Some advocate placing

---

Box 1. Tools for laparoendoscopic gastric surgery

Laparoscopic equipment
Laparoscopic monitors with picture-in-picture capabilities
Split-leg operating table
5–12 mm trocars
    Radially dilating trocars (Step-System, Tyco Healthcare,
        Princeton, New Jersey)
    2 mm needlescopic trocars (Imagyn Medical Technologies,
        Irvine, California)
    5 mm balloon-tipped trocars (Entec, Madison, Connecticut)
5 mm angled laparoscope
Laparoscopic injection needle
Laparoscopic ultrasonography
Laparoscopic instruments
    Hook
    Ultrasonic dissector
    Graspers
    Scissors
    Needle drivers
    Endoscopic staplers
    Seam Guard (GoreTex, Flagstaff, Arizona)
5 or 7 in, 22 gauge spinal needles
Endoloop
2-0 suture on SH needle

Endoscopic equipment
Videoendoscope
Esophageal overtube
Endoscopic injection needle
Dilute (1:100,000) epinephrine
Biopsy forceps
Endoscopic snare

---

a bowel clamp across the proximal small bowel, or using a balloon-tipped nasogastric tube to avoid bowel distension; however, the authors have not found small bowel distension to be a problem if inflation is only added as needed by the endoscopist.

Several trocars are available for securing intragastric access (see Box 1). The radially dilating trocars work through a sheath initially passed into the stomach over a Veress needle. The sheath expands as the working trocar is placed through it. If needed, a single gastric seromuscular suture can be placed at the gastric entrance site to prevent the stomach from slipping away from the anterior abdominal wall after trocar deployment. This suture is

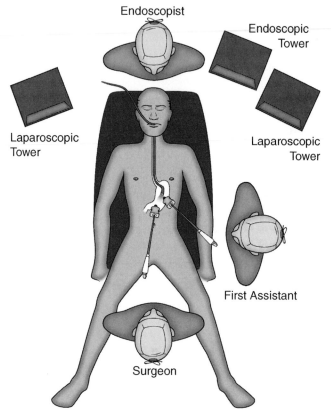

Fig. 1. Patient positioning and operating room set up for laparoscopic intragastric surgery. (Courtesy of Heather Sullivan.)

brought out through a small skin puncture using a laparoscopic suture passer, and secured at the skin level using a hemostat. This provides adequate stomach wall apposition with the anterior abdominal wall, and prevents retraction and resultant air leaks during insufflation. Alternatively, several trocars with various phalanges and balloon tips are available. The balloons/phalanges are inflated after penetrating the gastric wall, and provide internal fixation of the gastric wall to the anterior abdomen while maintaining gastric insufflation and preventing leakage of gastric contents. Others place large (22–24 French) percutaneous endoscopic gastrostomy (PEG) tubes for intragastric access; 5 mm trocars can be placed through these. Depending on the procedure, one to three trocars are usually necessary. When first performing an intragastric resection, the authors recommend using the 5 mm laparoscope as the operative camera, instead of the flexible videoendoscope for vision. We frequently use the video-endoscope, but it often has left-right inversion that increases the technical difficulties of the procedure. After obtaining intragastric access, we routinely inject dilute epinephrine (1:100,000), either through a laparoscopic port, the endoscope, or percutaneously with a long (5 or 7 in), 22 gauge spinal needle, to aid in maintaining adequate hemostasis and in identifying the correct dissection plane.

The details of the various procedures are discussed individually below. When necessary, intragastric sutures on SH needles can be delivered and removed transorally using the flexible endoscope through an esophageal overtube, or they can be skied and placed through a 5 mm port. Excised lesions are placed in an endoscopic retrieval bag and removed transorally. If endoscopic stapling devices are necessary, a 12 mm trocar is required.

At the conclusion of the procedure, the stomach is desufflated and the ports are returned to an intraperitoneal position. The gastrotomies are then repaired with an endoscopic stapler or sutures that are tied intracorporeally. A nasogastric tube is placed and left overnight. On postoperative day 1, a gastrograffin swallow is performed and the patient's diets is advanced.

Transgastric resection of early gastric cancer

Early gastric cancer is defined as lesions histologically confined to the mucosa and submucosa. Due to vigorous endoscopic screening in Japan, early gastric cancer comprises as many as 20% to 40% of gastric cancers in these series. The critical aspect in the management of these patients who have early gastric cancer is determining which patients are at risk for lymph node metastasis, and thus require more extensive surgery. Endosonography plays a pivotal role in selecting the appropriate surgical resection for these patients. Up to 15% of early gastric cancers invading the submucosal layer will have lymph node involvement and require more extensive resections [2]. Japanese investigators have determined that mucosal lesions less than 3 cm with superficial elevated or depressed features can undergo local mucosal resection because of the negligible chance of lymphatic spread [3]. The rarity of these lesions in Western series, and perhaps the difference in Japanese and Western pathologists' definition of early gastric cancer, should lead to a cautious interpretation of the Japanese data before translating their results to the treatment of gastric cancer among Western surgeons. To date, no Western trials exist evaluating the outcomes of intragastric treatment for early gastric cancer, and thus the only available literature to evaluate this approach reflects the Japanese experience.

Several minimally invasive options are available for the treatment of early gastric cancers. Flexible endoscopic methods are available to perform mucosal resection. Recent advances in endoscopic mucosal resection techniques, including the insulated-tip electrosurgical knife, have enabled en-bloc endoscopic resection of early-stage gastric cancers with reduced recurrence rates [4,5]. These improvements in endoscopic surgery have limited the widespread use of other techniques for resecting these tumors; however, certain lesions, particularly those located at the GE junction, fundus, and posterior wall of the stomach, are technically challenging for performing endoscopic mucosal resection. In addition, lesions larger than 1.5 cm often require piecemeal resection, and are a major cause of local recurrence in endoscopic series [3,4]. For these lesions, a laparoendoluminal approach is preferred. Current accepted indications for intragastric laparoscopic mucosal resection include: mucosal carcinoma difficult to completely resect using endoscopic mucosal resection; mucosal carcinoma of the elevated type less than 25 mm, or depressed type less than 15 mm; and mucosal carcinoma located anywhere in the stomach other than the anterior wall [1,6].

Realizing the advantages of an intragastric mucosal resection of early gastric cancer in those patients who were not candidates for an endoscopic approach, Ohashi [1] developed laparoscopic intraluminal gastric surgery in 1995. This technique enables preservation of the majority of the stomach; avoids postgastrectomy syndromes in patients who likely do not require extensive resections for cure; and provides a quick, less painful recovery than standard open surgery. He performed intragastric resection using three trocars placed through the abdominal wall into the gastric lumen in six patients who had early gastric cancer (Fig. 2). Four lesions were located on the posterior gastric wall, and one lesion each in the antrum and cardia. The lesions ranged in size from 1.5 to 2.5 cm. Ohashi used laparoendoscopic techniques to perform mucosal-based resections of all lesions, with laser cauterization of the remaining mucosal margin and muscular layer. In this series, no intraoperative or postoperative complications were reported. Mean operative time was 105 minutes, and there were no conversions to open surgery. Patients resumed oral intake within 2 to 3 days, and were discharged on average in 5 days. With a mean follow-up of 9 months, no patient experienced recurrence of gastric cancer.

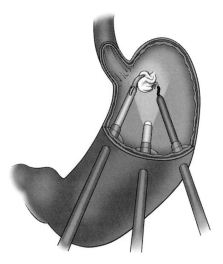

Fig. 2. Laparoscopic intragastric surgery for early gastric cancer.

Based on this encouraging data, Ohgami and colleagues [7] reported the largest series of laparoscopic intragastric surgical resections for early gastric cancer in 17 patients, using a similar technique to that of Ohashi. The average size of the lesion treated in this series was 9 mm (range 5–25 mm). The technical demands of this procedure were evident in the average operative times of over 4 hours. Despite these challenges, the study authors reported no intraoperative complications or conversions to an open procedure. Three patients developed mild postoperative stenosis at the cardia that required endoscopic balloon dilation. Complete follow-up was obtained in all patients for an average of 35 months. The study authors reported one local recurrence from a lesion located at the cardia, 2 years after resection. This was another small early cancer that was successfully treated with endoscopic laser ablation. The remaining patients were all alive and free of disease.

Recently, Kobayashi and coworkers [8] reported their long-term experience with laparoscopic intragastric mucosal resection for early gastric cancer. During the 4-year study period, these authors performed 350 gastric resections for cancer, and attempted laparoscopic intragastric surgery on seven highly selected patients who had early gastric cancer. The lesions averaged 1 cm in diameter and were located along the lesser curvature or posterior gastric wall. The average operative time was 210 minutes. Even in these highly selected patients, four (57%) conversions to an open procedure were necessary due to intraoperative hemorrhage (n = 3). Additionally, one patient required full-thickness resection; intragastric insufflation could not be maintained and the procedure was converted. Of significant concern, one patient who had a positive surgical margin that was initially felt to be a cautery effect subsequently developed a mucosal stump recurrence at 28 months after resection, and was managed with a distal gastrectomy. With an average follow-up of 8 years, these authors reported no other recurrence. Based on the high conversion rate and the one local recurrence (14%), the study authors no longer prefer laparoscopic intragastric approaches, and favor open local resection for those lesions that are not amenable to laparoscopic wedge resection.

To overcome some of the technical difficulties of laparoscopic intragastric surgery, Yamashita and colleagues [9] described an alternative access technique to perform intragastric surgery. They used a modified Buess technique, with similar instrumentation as used by transanal endoscopic microsurgeons, to perform transgastrostomal endoscopic surgery. This technique involves a 4 cm midline laparotomy. The stomach is then delivered into the wound and sutured to the skin edges. A full-thickness gastrotomy is performed and a 40 mm operative rectoscope is inserted over the resection area. Special Buess-type endoscopic equipment is used to perform the resection.

Advantages of this technique included the avoidance of CO_2 insufflation of the stomach, enabling full-thickness resection when necessary, and requiring only one gastrotomy instead of the three required for intragastric surgery. In their initial experience, the study authors reported six patients undergoing resection of early small carcinomas: four located on the lesser curvature and one each located on the posterior and anterior gastric walls. The tumors averaged 2.0 cm. The average operative time was 148 minutes. With an average of 13 months follow-up, no recurrences have been identified. Similarly, Nakagoe and coworkers [10] reported no episodes of local recurrence at an average of 5 years after using this approach in five patients who had early gastric cancer.

Although published series of laparoscopic intragastric resection of early gastric cancer mainly include case series (Table 1) [1,7–12], according to a survey of the Japan Society for Endoscopic Surgery, almost 260 intragastric mucosal resections were performed in Japan between 1992 and 2001 [13]. These responders had self-reported intraoperative and postoperative complication rates of 4.2% and 6.5%, respectively. Although this technically demanding procedure is still in its infancy and further long term follow-up with particular attention to cancer recurrence is necessary, it seems a viable option for the treatment of early gastric cancer in appropriately selected patients.

Transgastric management of gastrointestinal stromal tumors

Gastrointestinal stromal tumors (GISTs) are rare tumors with an annual incidence of four per million persons [14]. Typically these tumors are incidentally identified in patients undergoing upper endoscopy for unrelated complaints. With more advanced tumors, patients can present with bleeding, abdominal pain, weight loss, and a palpable mass. Although GISTs can be found throughout the gastrointestinal tract, the stomach is the predominant site, accounting for 52% of GISTS in one large series [15]. Of GISTs within the stomach, almost 80% are located within the fundus or body [16]. Given the submucosal nature of these tumors, endoscopic biopsies are notoriously inaccurate. Endoscopic ultrasound provides the critical information needed to define the relationship of the tumor to the layers of the gastric wall. Under the guidance of endoscopic ultrasound, fine-needle aspiration can be performed along with immunohistochemical analysis to improve diagnostic accuracy to 78% to 91% [17]. Other radiologic imaging tools, including CT scan and MRI, are useful in evaluating metastatic spread.

GISTs are derived from the pacemaker cells of the gastrointestinal tract identified as the interstitial cells of Cajal [18]. Previously these tumors were thought to arise from the smooth muscle cells of the gastrointestinal tract, and were classified as leiomyomas or leiomyosarcomas. With improvements in immunohistochemical analysis, these tumors have been found to express several cellular markers, including CD-117, a marker of the c-kit gene product, and CD-34, a human progenitor cell antigen [14]. Lymphatic

Table 1
Laparoscopic intragastric management of early gastric cancer

Study	Patients (N)	Technique	Tumor diameter (cm)	Complications (N)	Conversions (N)	OR time (min)	LOS (Days)	Recurrence (N)	Followup (m)
Ohashi [1]	6	Intragastric	2.3	0	0	105	5	0	9
Shimizu et al [11]	4	Intragastric	2.3	1 (bleeding)	1	298	16	-	-
Kobayasi et al [8]	7	Intragastric	4.0	4 (bleeding)	4 (bleeding)	210	12	1	96
Yamashita et al [9]	6	Transgastrostomal	2.0	0	0	148	9	0	11
Nakagoe et al [10]	5	Transgastrostomal	2.4	1 (bleeding GU) away from OR site	0	135	-	0	64
Oghami et al [7]	17	Intragastric	0.9	3 (cardia stenosis) postop	0	245	8	1	35
Watanabe et al [12]	4	Transgastrostomal	1.7	Positive surgical margin	1	120	9	0	11

Abbreviations: GU, gastric ulcer; LOS, length of stay; N, number; OR, operating room.

involvement of GISTs is uncommon, as with other sarcomas; therefore formal lymphadenectomy is not part of the standard surgical resection. Complete surgical resection of the primary tumor with a simple negative margin is the only definitive therapy for cure. These tumors can be resected by laparotomy, laparoscopy, or by using endoluminal techniques. The improved exposure of the upper abdomen during laparoscopy, the fact that a formal lymph node dissection is not necessary for the treatment of these tumors, and the extensive experience with exposure and manipulation of the stomach laparoscopically for fundoplication and other procedures have enabled the application of a minimally invasive approach to the resection of these tumors.

The authors offer the minimally invasive approach to the majority of our patients. The operative technique is tailored to the tumor location. For tumors located on the anterior gastric wall, the lesser and greater curvature, we prefer a laparoscopic wedge resection. Those lesions located on the posterior gastric wall can be treated by full mobilization of the greater curve of the stomach, with wedge resection or a large anterior gastrotomy and resection inside the stomach. Those lesions near the GE junction or pylorus are typically not amenable to a laparoscopic wedge resection because of inaccessibility, the fear of stricture formation at the gastric inlet or outlet, or the possibility of inducing severe reflux. An open approach to these tumors requires either a gastrectomy, or in the case of a GE junction lesion, an esophagogastrectomy. In the setting of a potentially benign lesion and those that require a simple negative margin, the morbidity and postoperative quality of life from these major resections can be unacceptably poor. In this setting, and for some posterior gastric tumors, the authors have offered an endoluminal laparoscopic resection. Full-thickness resections can be performed using this technique—a submucosal resection is often all that is needed; however, they are also more technically demanding because gas insufflation of the stomach is difficult to maintain.

Peritoneal access is gained through the umbilicus. An initial diagnostic laparoscopy is performed to rule out peritoneal seeding or hepatic metastasis. Intraoperative ultrasound is used to evaluate the liver for metastatic deposits and the primary tumor for its relationship with the gastric wall and surrounding structures. Two to three transgastric trocars are placed as previously described. A dilute epinephrine solution is injected around the tumor as a tumescent to aid in dissection of the submucosal plane and to decrease bleeding. The lesion is enucleated from the submucosal-muscular junction using an electrocautery hook at very low wattage. Typically, the mucosal defect is closed with intragastric suturing techniques. The mass can be removed transorally with the flexible endoscope.

The effectiveness and safety of the laparoendoscopic treatment of GISTs of the stomach has been documented in several series (Table 2) [19–26]. Although the majority of these reports are composed of primarily case reports and small series, the initial outcomes are encouraging. In properly

Table 2
Laparoscopic endoluminal resection of gastrointestinal stromal tumors

Study	Patients (N)	Tumor size (cm)	Tumor location	OR time (minutes)	LOS (days)	Conversion (N)	Complications (N)	Recurrence (N)	Followup (months)
Sekimoto et al [19]	1	2	EG junction	-	-	0	0	0	1
Heniford et al [20]	1	4	EG junction	135	3	0	0	0	9
Choi and Oh [21]	9	-	Posterior wall	140	6	0	0	0	32 maximum
Ludwig et al [22]	8	2.5	Posterior wall	67	10.2	1	1 (post-wall perforation converted)	0	15
Nguyen et al [23]	1	2.8	EG junction	180	3	0	0	0	9
Pross et al [24]	5	3.4	EG junction	80–105	4–7	0	0	-	-
Walsh et al [25]	13	3.8	EG junction 8 Posterior wall 4 Fundus 1	186	3.8	0	0	0	16.2
Uchikoshi et al [26]	7	4.3	EG junction	141	6	1 (required full thickness resection)	0	1 (local recurrence 2 years postop)	12–96

selected patients, conversions rates have ranged from 0% to 5%, and conversions have primarily been when full-thickness resections are required. Major operative or postoperative morbidity has not been reported. Long-term follow-up is only available in a few series (1 month to 8 years), and local recurrence has only been reported in one case at 2 years post-operatively. Long-term clinical outcomes will most likely be determined by tumor biology [27,28]; however, in the absence of prospective randomized trials comparing minimally invasive techniques and conventional open techniques for the treatment of GISTs, definitive conclusions about the perioperative, immunologic, and oncologic advantages of this approach cannot be drawn. The only available long-term follow-up retrospectively comparing laparoscopic and open resections for GISTs tumors was reported by Matthews and colleagues [27]. These authors noted a significant reduction in postoperative hospitalization in the laparoscopic group. Interestingly, recurrence rates were similar between the two groups; with an average of 1.6 years of follow-up, one patient each in the laparoscopic and open groups died of metastatic disease.

The largest experience of laparoendoscopic resection of GIST tumors was recently reported by Walsh and coworkers [25]. During a 40-month period, these authors resected 14 gastric stromal tumors in 13 patients using endoluminal intragastric techniques. The majority of these lesions were located at or near the GE junction. The advantages of the minimally invasive approach were apparent in the early postoperative recovery (average length of stay of 3.8 days) and the absence of intraoperative or postoperative morbidity in these patients who would have otherwise required an esophagogastrectomy. Given the expertise of this group, 3 patients required full-thickness excision and were completed using endolaparoscopic techniques; however, the study authors do note that full-thickness excision increases the technical demands of the procedure. With complete follow-up in all patients for a mean of 16 months, they identified no clinical or endoscopic recurrence.

GISTs are a rare group of neoplasms that are being increasing identified early in otherwise asymptomatic patients. The appropriate surgical approach for these patients is continuing to develop. For those lesions located near the gastroesophageal junction or on the posterior gastric wall, an increasing number of combined laparoscopic and endoscopic resections are being performed. This approach offers these patients a curative resection avoiding the significant morbidity of open segmental resections of the stomach.

Transgastric pancreatic pseudocyst drainage

Acute pancreatitis and chronic pancreatitis with an acute exacerbation can result in disruption of the pancreatic ductal system, pancreatic enzymatic leakage, and pseudocyst formation. This collection of pancreatic fluid is typically enclosed by a fibrous wall of inflammatory tissue that forms adjacent to peripancreatic tissue in the lesser sac. Symptomatic, persistent, acute pseudocysts present longer than 6 weeks typically require drainage, because spontaneous resolution is rare and complication rates increase dramatically [29]. Chronic pseudocysts larger than 6 cm also require drainage. Because of the perceived morbidity of standard open surgical drainage of pseudocysts via laparotomy, several less invasive treatments have been described. Increasing numbers of these cases have been reported, and some authors have challenged the standard dictum of open surgical drainage of pancreatic pseudocysts. Percutaneous external drainage by interventional radiologists and endoscopic internal drainage by gastroenterologists have been frequently described, but the techniques are limited by the small orifice created for pseudocyst drainage. Alternatively, a variety of laparoscopic approaches to the surgical drainage of pseudocysts that maintain the minimally invasive approach while providing wide drainage, similar to drainage as performed in open surgery, have been reported.

Percutaneous radiologic drainage of pseudocysts is inexpensive and can be performed under local anesthesia. Catheter-related complications occur in up to 10% of patients, however; typically at least 2 to 3 weeks of external drainage is necessary in highly selected patients, and unsuccessful drainage can result in difficult-to-manage pancreaticocutaneous fistulas or infected pseudocysts [30–32]. Several large series have reported recurrence rates of as much as to 22% to 23%, despite prolonged drainage [31,33–35]. Endoscopists have also entered the realm of minimally invasive internal drainage of pseudocysts. Both transpapillary stents and transmural drainage techniques have been described. Some pseudocysts in which a communication to the main pancreatic duct can be demonstrated with endoscopic retrograde cholangiopancreatography (ERCP) may benefit from transpapillary stenting in the setting of ampullary stenosis or inflammatory stricture, by effectively relieving the high pressure locus; however, the occurrence of secondary infection of the pseudocyst, stent clogging, pancreatic duct inflammation, stricture formation, and recurrence rates secondary to inadequate communication between the pseudocyst and enteric cavity have limited the success of these techniques [36].

Surgical drainage of pseudocysts remains the standard to which other methods must be compared [37]. Traditionally this has required a laparotomy, with the associated risks in these typically compromised patients. Standard open approaches have reported operative morbidity rates of 10% to 30%, mortality rates of 1% to 5%, and recurrence rates of 5% to 20% [38,39]. These limitations have fostered the previously mentioned attempts at other less-invasive drainage procedures, procedures that have decreased the operative morbidity at the cost of potentially higher recurrence rates secondary to inadequate drainage techniques. The introduction of laparoscopic surgery in the treatment of pancreatic disease has enabled a minimally invasive approach that maintains the open surgical principles of pseudocysts drainage, including creation of wide and dependent communication between the pseudocyst and the appropriate bowel lumen, debridement of the pseudocyst cavity, and biopsy of the pseudocyst wall. Minimally invasive techniques for pseudocyst drainage can be tailored based on the location of the pseudocyst. Options include Roux-en-Y pseudocyst-jejunostomy, pseudocyst-duodenostomy, and pseudocyst-gastrostomy.

When surgical drainage is indicated, pancreatic pseudocysts adherent to the posterior gastric wall are best drained by pseudocyst-gastrostomy [40]. This can be approached laparoscopically through a large anterior gastrotomy or through the lesser sac [41]. Alternatively, an endoluminal transgastric approach can be used. This technique was initially described in 1993 and is summarized below [42].

Patient setup and initial transgastric access are similar to other endoluminal procedures as previously described. Depending on the technique for creation of the pseudocystgastrostomy, various size and numbers of ports can be used. If the gastroscope is used for visualization, one transgastric port can be used to complete the procedure, but two allow for suction, suturing, and so forth. If endoscopic staplers are used for the pseudocyst-gastrostomy, then, as previously mentioned, a 12 mm trocar is necessary. In most cases, the pseudocyst can be seen bulging into the posterior gastric lumen; otherwise, it can be localized with endoscopic or laparoscopic ultrasonography. Typically, a long aspirating 18 or 22 gauge needle is passed through the laparoscopic port or directly through the abdominal wall of the stomach to confirm the cavity location. Confirmation using either the endoscopic ultrasound or review of the preoperative imaging is critical to assure the absence of large vessels within the pseudocyst wall at the site of entrance into the pseudocyst wall. The pseudocyst cavity is entered through the posterior wall of the stomach, using the harmonic dissector or electrocautery. A biopsy of the pseudocyst wall is obtained and sent for pathologic examination, and the necrotic debris is removed. A large-diameter communication (at least 4 cm) is created with the endoscopic stapler, cautery, or ultrasonic dissector, with or without intracorporeal suturing techniques (Fig. 3). Postoperative hemorrhage at the anastomotic site has been reported, typically when a stapler or electrocautery alone is used for the anastomosis. The authors typically use an endoscopic stapler reinforced with Seam Guard, and we have not encountered postoperative hemorrhage in our experience. The transgastric ports are then removed to an intraperitoneal position and the gastrotomies are either stapled closed or oversewn.

Transgastric pseudocystgastrostomy was first described in 1993 by Atabek and colleagues [42]. They used a percutaneous endoscopic gastrostomy tube as a working port and the flexible endoscope as an operating camera. They performed a 1.5 cm pseudocyst gastrostomy, which recurred and subsequently required a repeated minimally invasive procedure for complete drainage. To date, approximately 40 cases of transgastric

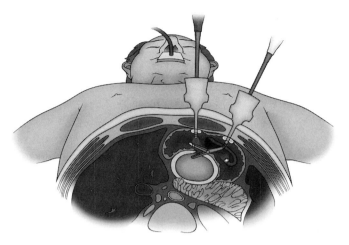

Fig. 3. Laparoscopic intragastric stapled pseudocystgastrostomy.

endoluminal pseudocyst drainage have been reported in the literature (Table 3) [36,41–45]. In this combined experience, the mean operative time was 123 minutes and the average length of stay was 4.6 days. Two patients were converted to an open procedure. One conversion was caused by lack of adherence of the pseudocyst wall to the posterior stomach, and another was secondary to uncontrollable hemorrhage from the pseudocyst wall. Four major complications occurred. Mori and coworkers [46] reported two cases of uncontrollable hemorrhage from the pseudocyst wall during the use of electrocautery to perform the posterior pseudocystgastrotomy. They noted that a retrospective review of the preoperative CT and MRI revealed large vessels running between the pseudocyst and gastric walls. Other authors have advocated the use of intraoperative endoscopic ultrasound to evaluate the presence and location of vessels within the pseudocyst wall before performing the gastrotomy incision [36]. This underscores the importance of appropriate patient selection and careful review of preoperative radiologic imaging. Park and Heniford [41] also reported two cases of postoperative bleeding after intragastric pseudocystgastrostomy requiring blood transfusion; both cases had been stapled without reinforcement. They now advocate applying sutures to the anastomosis to ensure adequate hemostasis. In other studies, with 6 to 32 months of radiologic follow-up, two pseudocyst recurrences have been reported [42,43]. Both of these recurrences occurred early in the respective authors' experience because of a small incision made for the pseudocystgastrostomy. In one case the pseudocyst became infected, requiring subsequent open surgical drainage.

Intragastric pseudocystgastrostomy is a minimally invasive technique that bridges the wide gap between interventional and endoscopic drainage techniques and open surgical drainage [43]. It accomplishes these goals by providing concomitant creation of wide dependent pseudocyst enterostomy

Table 3
Laparoscopic endoluminal pseudocyst drainage

Study	Patients	Mean OR time (min)	Mean LOS (days)	Conversion (N)	Pseudocyst resolution (%)	Complication (%)	Follow-up (months)	Recurrence (%)
Mori et al [43]	18	-	8.6	4	94	17	6–32	6
Chowbey et al [44]	5	90	3.0	0	100	0	6	0
Ramachandran et al [36]	5	110	4	0	100	0	12	0
Attabek et al [42]	1	-		0	100	-	-	100
Park et al [41]	16	150	3.3	1 (gastric varices)	100	13	15.8	0
Ammori et al [45]	3	165	4	0	100	0	6	0

communication, and pancreatic debridement, while avoiding many of the shortcomings of other minimally invasive drainage techniques (endoscopic and percutaneous). These include obstruction of drainage communication, tract infections, bleeding, and pancreaticocutaneous fistulas. With the short- to mid-term follow-up available, this laparoscopic endoluminal technique appears to be favorable. Because open principles are maintained, it seems that recurrence rates should not be different. Based on the available data, pseudocyst resolution seems equal to that of other open series. Further long-term data are awaited before this technically demanding procedure can be fully endorsed.

Summary

Laparoendoluminal techniques are the next frontier in modern surgery. They provide a minimally invasive approach to gastric diseases that enables organ preservation while maintaining open surgical principles. Laparoscopic direct access to the stomach provides a magnified, high-resolution image for precise excision using widely available laparoscopic instrumentation [47]. Further improvements in flexible endoscopic equipment, combined with the infusion of robotic instrumentation, will aid in overcoming the technical demands of this procedure and fuel the growth of endoluminal gastric surgery. Based on the currently available data, in appropriately selected patients, endoluminal gastric surgery affords the patients a definitive surgical procedure with all the advantages of a minimally invasive approach.

References

[1] Ohashi S. Laparoscopic intraluminal (intragastric) surgery for early gastric cancer. A new concept in laparoscopic surgery. Surg Endosc 1995;9:169–71.
[2] Cuschieri A. Laparoscopic gastric resection. Surg Clin North Am 2000;80:1269–84;viii.
[3] Ono H, Kondo H, Gotoda T, et al. Endoscopic mucosal resection for treatment of early gastric cancer. Gut 2001;48:225–9.
[4] Makuuchi H, Kise Y, Shimada H, et al. Endoscopic mucosal resection for early gastric cancer. Semin Surg Oncol 1999;17:108–16.
[5] Miyamoto S, et al. A new technique for endoscopic mucosal resection with an insulated-tip electrosurgical knife improves the completeness of resection of intramucosal gastric neoplasms. Gastrointest Endosc 2002;55:576–81.
[6] Kitano S, Shiraishi N. Current status of laparoscopic gastrectomy for cancer in Japan. Surg Endosc 2004;18:182–5.
[7] Ohgami M, Otani Y, Kumai K, et al. Curative laparoscopic surgery for early gastric cancer: five years experience. World J Surg 1999;23:187–92 [discussion: 192–3].
[8] Kobayashi T, Kazui T, Kimura T. Surgical local resection for early gastric cancer. Surg Laparosc Endosc Percutan Tech 2003;13:299–303.
[9] Yamashita Y, Maekawa T, Sakai T, et al. Transgastrostomal endoscopic surgery for early gastric carcinoma and submucosal tumor. Surg Endosc 1999;13:361–4.
[10] Nakagoe T, Tanaka K, Yasutake T, et al. Long-term outcomes of intragastric endoscopic mucosal resection using a modified buess technique for early gastric cancer. Dig Surg 2003;20:141–7.

[11] Shimizu S, Noshiro H, Nagai E, et al. Laparoscopic gastric surgery in a Japanese institution: analysis of the initial 100 procedures. J Am Coll Surg 2003;197:372–8.

[12] Watanabe Y, Sato M, Kikkawa H, et al. Intragastric endoscopic mucosal resection through a temporary gastrostomy for early gastric cancer: usefulness of Buess-type endoscope. Eur J Surg 2001;167:362–5.

[13] Kitano S, Bandoh T, Kawano K. Endoscopic surgery in Japan. Minim Invasive Ther Allied Technol 2001;10:215–9.

[14] Miettinen M, Sarlomo-Rikala M, Lasota J. Gastrointestinal stromal tumors: recent advances in understanding of their biology. Hum Pathol 1999;30:1213–20.

[15] Emory TS, Sobin LH, Lukes L, et al. Prognosis of gastrointestinal smooth-muscle (stromal) tumors: dependence on anatomic site. Am J Surg Pathol 1999;23:82–7.

[16] Welch JP. Smooth muscle tumors of the stomach. Am J Surg 1975;130:279–85.

[17] Ando N, Goto H, Niwa Y, et al. The diagnosis of GI stromal tumors with EUS-guided fine needle aspiration with immunohistochemical analysis. Gastrointest Endosc 2002;55:37–43.

[18] Vanderwinden JM. Role of interstitial cells of Cajal and their relationship with the enteric nervous system. Eur J Morphol 1999;37:250–6.

[19] Sekimoto M, Tamura S, Hasuike Y, et al. A new technique for laparoscopic resection of a submucosal tumor on the posterior wall of the gastric fundus. Surg Endosc 1999;13:71–4.

[20] Heniford BT, Arca MJ, Walsh RM. The mini-laparoscopic intragastric resection of a gastroesophageal stromal tumor: a novel approach. Surg Laparosc Endosc Percutan Tech 2000;10:82–5.

[21] Choi YB, Oh ST. Laparoscopy in the management of gastric submucosal tumors. Surg Endosc 2000;14:741–5.

[22] Ludwig K, Wilhelm L, Scharlau U, et al. Laparoscopic-endoscopic rendezvous resection of gastric tumors. Surg Endosc 2002;16:1561–5.

[23] Nguyen NT, Jim J, Nguyen A, et al. Laparoscopic resection of gastric stromal tumor: a tailored approach. Am Surg 2003;69:946–50.

[24] Pross M, Wolff S, Nestler G, et al. A technique for endo-organ resection of gastric wall tumors using one intragastric trocar. Endoscopy 2003;35:613–5.

[25] Walsh RM, Ponsky J, Brody F, et al. Combined endoscopic/laparoscopic intragastric resection of gastric stromal tumors. J Gastrointest Surg 2003;7:386–92.

[26] Uchikoshi F, Ito T, Nishida T, et al. Laparoscopic intragastric resection of gastric stromal tumor located at the esophago-cardiac junction. Surg Laparosc Endosc Percutan Tech 2004; 14:1–4.

[27] Matthews BD, Walsh RM, Kercher KW, et al. Laparoscopic vs open resection of gastric stromal tumors. Surg Endosc 2002;16:803–7.

[28] Trupiano JK, Stewart RE, Misick C, et al. Gastric stromal tumors: a clinicopathologic study of 77 cases with correlation of features with nonaggressive and aggressive clinical behaviors. Am J Surg Pathol 2002;26:705–14.

[29] Bradley EL, Clements JL Jr, Gonzalez AC. The natural history of pancreatic pseudocysts: a unified concept of management. Am J Surg 1979;137:135–41.

[30] Heider R, Meyer AA, Galanko JA, et al. Percutaneous drainage of pancreatic pseudocysts is associated with a higher failure rate than surgical treatment in unselected patients. Ann Surg 1999;229:781–7 [discussion: 787–9].

[31] Spivak H, Galloway JR, Amerson JR, et al. Management of pancreatic pseudocysts. J Am Coll Surg 1998;186:507–11.

[32] vanSonnenberg E, Wittich GR, Casola G, et al. Percutaneous drainage of infected and noninfected pancreatic pseudocysts: experience in 101 cases. Radiology 1989;170:757–61.

[33] Freeny PC. Percutaneous management of pancreatic fluid collections. Baillieres Clin Gastroenterol 1992;6:259–72.

[34] Grosso M, Gandini G, Cassinis MC, et al. Percutaneous treatment (including pseudocystogastrostomy) of 74 pancreatic pseudocysts. Radiology 1989;173:493–7.

[35] Gumaste UV, Dave PB. Pancreatic pseudocyst drainage—the needle or the scalpel? J Clin Gastroenterol 1991;13:500–5.

[36] Ramachandran CS, Goel D, Arora V, et al. Gastroscopic-assisted laparoscopic cystogastrostomy in the management of pseudocysts of the pancreas. Surg Laparosc Endosc Percutan Tech 2002;12:433–6.

[37] Bhattacharya D, Ammori BJ. Minimally invasive approaches to the management of pancreatic pseudocysts: review of the literature. Surg Laparosc Endosc Percutan Tech 2003; 13:141–8.

[38] Huibregtse K, Schneider B, Vrij AA, et al. Endoscopic pancreatic drainage in chronic pancreatitis. Gastrointest Endosc 1988;34:9–15.

[39] Kohler H, Schafmayer A, Ludtke FE, et al. Surgical treatment of pancreatic pseudocysts. Br J Surg 1987;74:813–5.

[40] Grace PA, Williamson RC. Modern management of pancreatic pseudocysts. Br J Surg 1993; 80:573–81.

[41] Park AE, Heniford BT. Therapeutic laparoscopy of the pancreas. Ann Surg 2002;236: 149–58.

[42] Atabek U, Mayer D, Amin A, et al. Pancreatic cystogastrostomy by combined upper endoscopy and percutaneous transgastric instrumentation. J Laparoendosc Surg 1993;3: 501–4.

[43] Mori T, Abe N, Sugiyama M, et al. Laparoscopic pancreatic cystgastrostomy. J Hepatobiliary Pancreat Surg 2002;9:548–54.

[44] Chowbey PK, Soni V, Sharma A, et al. Laparoscopic intragastric stapled cystogastrostomy for pancreatic pseudocyst. J Laparoendosc Adv Surg Tech A 2001;11:201–5.

[45] Ammori BJ, Bhattacharya D, Senapati PS. Laparoscopic endogastric pseudocyst gastrostomy: a report of three cases. Surg Laparosc Endosc Percutan Tech 2002;12:437–40.

[46] Mori T, Abe N, Sugiyama M, et al. Laparoscopic pancreatic cystgastrostomy. J Hepatobiliary Pancreat Surg 2000;7:28–34.

[47] Mittal SK, Filipi CJ. Indications for endo-organ gastric excision. Surg Endosc 2000;14: 318–25.

ELSEVIER
SAUNDERS

SURGICAL
CLINICS OF
NORTH AMERICA

Surg Clin N Am 85 (2005) 1009–1020

Limited Gastric Resection

Jeffrey D. Wayne, MD[a],*, Richard H. Bell, Jr, MD[b]

[a]Division of Surgical Oncology, Northwestern University Feinberg School of Medicine,
Galter 3-150, 201 East Huron Street, Chicago, IL 60611, USA
[b]Department of Surgery, Northwestern University Feinberg School of Medicine,
Galter 3-150, 201 East Huron Street, Chicago, IL 60611, USA

Although the incidence and death rates of gastric carcinoma have declined since 1930, in 2004 there were still expected to be 22,710 new cases diagnosed and 11,780 deaths from this disease in the United States alone [1]. Furthermore, despite advances in our understanding of the pathogenesis of this tumor, most cases present at a relatively advanced stage. This is reflected by the poor 5-year survival rates from gastric adenocarcinoma, which continue to hover at or below 20% [2]. Thus, there remains considerable controversy regarding the optimal management of these patients, who often have incurable disease. Specifically, debate remains regarding the extent of gastric resection as well as the extent of lymph node dissection. Although Japanese authors continue to promote extended gastric resections with regional nodal dissection, the success of such procedure in a Western population has yet to be validated. This article outlines the argument against extended or total gastrectomy for gastric cancer, and describes the current approach to other less common tumors of the stomach, which may often be treated by nonanatomic or limited gastric resection. The role of surgery in the palliation of patients who have Stage IV disease is outlined, and specific attention is given to gastric lymphoma, gastrointestinal stromal tumors (GIST), and gastric carcinoid tumors.

Extent of resection for gastric ulcer

R0 resection, defined as resection of all gross disease with microscopically negative margins, has been shown to have a clear impact upon overall

---

* Corresponding author.
E-mail address: jwayne@northwestern.edu (J.D. Wayne).

surgical.theclinics.com

survival after potentially curative surgery [3]. In the German Gastric Cancer Study, a prospective multicenter trial, the calculated 10-year survival rate in the entire population of patients who had gastric cancer was 26.3% versus 36.1% after an R0 resection [3]. Similarly, Hallissey and colleagues [4] found that 19% of patients enrolled in a large, multi-institution adjuvant therapy trial had an R1 resection or resection-line involvement. Only 9% of patients who had Stage I through III disease and a positive margin survived beyond 5 years, as compared with 27% for those undergoing R0 resection. Thus, the goal of any surgery for gastric cancer is the removal of all gross and microscopic disease. Given the propensity for submucosal spread of tumor, proximal margins of 5 to 6 cm, with routine frozen-section analysis, are considered optimal by many authors [5,6].

In an effort to lower the rate of positive margins, total gastrectomy has been proposed as the operation of choice for all operable gastric cancers. This approach was fostered by historical data from single institutions. There have now been at least three trials that have attempted to address this hypothesis [7–9]. Gouzi and coworkers [7] reported results from a pro-spective multicenter trial of elective total gastrectomy versus subtotal gastrectomy for adenocarcinoma of the antrum operated on with curative intent. Although elective total gastrectomy did not increase mortality in this series of 169 patients, it also did not improve the 5-year survival, which was 48% in both treatment arms. Similarly, Robertson and colleagues [8] randomized 55 patients who had antral cancer to either subtotal gas-trectomy or total gastrectomy with an extended lymph node dissection and en-bloc distal pancreatectomy and splenectomy. In their series, total gas-trectomy was associated with increased operative time, greater transfusion requirements, and longer hospital stay. Interestingly, median survival was significantly better in the subtotal gastrectomy group (1511 versus 922 days, $P < 0.05$). Finally, Bozzetti and coworkers [9] concluded that subtotal gastrectomy should be the procedure of choice for cancer of the distal half of the stomach, provided that a negative proximal margin can be adequately achieved. This assertion was made based on an equivalent 5-year survival probability for both groups in this study (65.3% for subtotal gastrectomy versus 62.4% for total gastrectomy).

Proximal gastric cancer

Adenocarcinoma of the gastric cardia and gastroesophageal junction (GEJ) appears to be a distinct clinical entity, as compared with distal gastric cancer [10]. Furthermore, with the incidence of proximal gastric cancer escalating across all races and age groups, it is imperative to understand the surgical options for these complex lesions [11]. For tumors originating from the distal esophagus, esophagectomy, either transabdominal with a cervical anastamosis or via the abdomen and right chest (Ivor-Lewis), is clearly the procedure of choice. In an effort to ascertain whether esophagogastrectomy would offer a survival advantage over total gastrectomy with an esophagojejunal anastomosis for tumors of the cardia, Rudiger Siewert and coworkers [12] reviewed their experience with 1002 patients who had adenocarcinoma of the esophagogastric junction. After dividing tumors into three types based on location of the tumor, demographic data and long-term survival were analyzed for cancers of the distal esophagus (Type I), cardia (Type II), and the subcardial fundus (Type III). In this study, operative mortality was higher for esophagectomy as compared with extended total gastrectomy. Furthermore, R0 resection and lymph node status were the dominant prognostic factors influencing survival in the study's multivariate analysis. Finally, in Type II lesions, the pattern of lymphatic spread was primarily to paracardial, lesser curvature, and left gastric nodes. These data in toto led the authors to recommend total gastrectomy over esophagectomy if a margin-negative resection can be achieved.

One alternative approach that has been reported for proximal gastric lesions is the proximal subtotal gastrectomy. Although no prospective studies have compared this method to total gastrectomy or transhiatal esophagogastrectomy for GE junction tumors, surgeons from Memorial Sloan Kettering Cancer Center have published their retrospective experience [13]. The study population consisted of 98 patients who underwent either total gastrectomy (TG) or proximal subtotal gastrectomy (PG) for proximal gastric cancer over a 10-year period. There were no differences between the groups in terms of morbidity, mortality, or 5-year survival (43% for PG versus 41% for TG, P = non-significant). It remains to be seen whether such excellent results can be achieved at other centers.

Thus to summarize, there is currently no evidence to support the routine performance of total gastrectomy for lesions of the distal fundus or antrum, so long as histologically negative margins can be achieved without compromising the gastric inlet. Thus, the authors' current practice is to perform a subtotal gastrectomy with Billroth II reconstruction for tumors of the distal stomach. We favor a total gastrectomy with Roux-en-Y esophagojejunostomy for most cancers of the fundus and proximal stomach, particularly if they are clear of the GEJ by 2 to 3 cm, or originate near the GEJ but extend along the lesser curve. For tumors of the cardia, within 1 to 2 cm of the GEJ, we perform either a transthoracic esophagogastrectomy or transhiatal esophagogastrectomy with gastric interposition. This approach is also adopted when there is evidence of significant lymphadenopathy along the distal esophagus on preoperative CT or endoscopic ultrasonography (EUS).

Palliative resection for gastric cancer

In patients found to have Stage IV disease by preoperative staging or at laparoscopy, attempts at radical R0 resection are usually abandoned; however, palliative procedures, either in the form of limited resection or bypass, may be indicated to relieve symptoms, control pain, or improve quality of life [14]. Traditionally, total gastrectomy was not considered an appropriate palliative procedure, due to the high rates of morbidity and mortality [15]. More recently, with advances in surgical technique, this dictum has been challenged and total gastrectomy has been performed in series of highly selected patients. Monson and coworkers reported a series of 53 patients from the Mayo Clinic who underwent total gastrectomy with palliative intent [16]. The decision to perform a total gastrectomy was based on tumor location in 30% of patients and on extent of disease in 70%. Seventeen percent of patients in this series were diagnosed with linitis plastica. The mortality in this series was a respectable 8%, and median survival was 19 months. A full 24% of these patients survived for 2 years. Perhaps most importantly, quality of life was graded good in 59% of patients and poor in only 13%. Most current series report results that are far less compelling, however. In reporting data from the Dutch Gastric Cancer Trial, Hartgrink and colleagues [17] noted that 285 patients were found to have incurable disease at laparotomy. Although overall survival was greater if a gastric resection was performed (8.1 versus 5.4 months, respectively), morbidity and mortality rates were high (50% and 20%, respectively). Similarly, Miner and coworkers [14] reported the experience of surgeons at the Memorial Sloan Kettering Cancer Center with patients who underwent a noncurative (R1/R2) resection for gastric cancer. Despite the fact that palliative operations less frequently included an esophageal anastamosis, and had less extensive lymphadenectomy, operative morbidity was 54% and mortality was 6%.

Although once only amenable only to open gastrojejunostomy, distal obstructions may now be alleviated by the endoscopic placement of self-expanding endoluminal stents [18]. Such stents have been effective in up to 85% of cases, with an average uninterrupted duration of function of 5 to 6 months. In one recent series [19], stent placement was successful in 100% of patients, with 97% of patients able to tolerate some form of oral intake. Perhaps more importantly, nonoperative approaches to gastric outlet obstruction allow patients who have Stage IV disease to proceed to palliative chemotherapy without delay. Because randomized clinical trials have suggested a benefit for chemotherapy versus best supportive care in patients who have Stage IV gastric cancer, this advantage is clinically meaningful [20]. Thus, whenever possible, patients who have M1 disease should be approached by nonoperative means. Gastric resection or bypass may have a role an occasional highly-selected patient; however, the high rates of morbidity and mortality, even in experienced hands, rarely justify a total or even distal gastrectomy.

Gastric lymphoma

Lymphomas of the stomach are the second most common gastric malignancy. Lymphomas of the stomach are of the non-Hodgkin's type, and in the United States compose 2% to 9% of malignancies of the stomach. The stomach is the most common site of extranodal non-Hodgkin's lymphoma (NHL), and accounts for nearly 50% of all such cases [21]. Presenting symptoms, like those of gastric adenocarcinoma, are nonspecific, and include loss of appetite, weight loss, vomiting, and bleeding. B symptoms (fever, night sweats) are relatively rare, and occurred in fewer than 12% of patients enrolled in a recent multicenter trial [22]. Risk factors for gastric lymphoma include *Helicobacter pylori* infection, immunosuppression after solid organ transplantation, celiac disease, inflammatory bowel disease, and HIV infection [23]. Diagnosis is most frequently made by endoscopy with biopsy. Staging studies include a complete blood count; lactate dehydrogenase and comprehensive chemistry panel; CT scans of the chest, abdomen and pelvis; and often a bone marrow biopsy. All pathology slides should be reviewed by an experienced hematopathologist [24].

Numerous staging systems have been used to stage gastrointestinal NHL, with the most commonly applied system being a modification of the Ann Arbor staging system for lymphoma [23]. For the surgeon, the most important determination is whether the NHL is confined to the stomach and perigastric nodes (Stages I and II), involves other intra-abdominal nodes and organs (Stage III), or exists beyond the abdomen (Stage IV) [25].

Over the past decade, the management of patients who have gastric lymphoma has undergone significant changes, with a shift away from surgical management, even in relatively localized (Stage I and II) cases [26]. Such changes have come about not only from the historic success of chemotherapy alone for more advanced (Stage III and IV) cases, but also from a better understanding of the etiology of gastric lymphoma [27]. Approximately 45% of all gastric lymphomas are low grade mucosa associated lymphoid tissue (MALT) lymphomas [22]. The gastric mucosa is normally devoid of lymphoid tissue. Thus, it is hypothesized that MALT develops in the stomach in response to chronic *H pylori* infection [28].

Patients who have low-grade MALT lymphomas usually present with Stage I or II disease and have an indolent course. Since the first report of regression of low-grade MALT lymphoma following eradication of *H pylori* in 1993, numerous trials [29] have documented the efficacy of such therapy, with complete remission rates between 50% and 100% [26]. In the German MALT Lymphoma Study [29], the complete remission rate was 81%; 9% of patients had only partial responses and 10% were nonresponders. More advanced low-grade lymphomas or those that do not regress with antibiotic therapy can be treated with combinations of *H pylori* eradication, radiation, or combination chemotherapy [30]. For localized persistent disease, modest doses of radiation, on the order of 30 Gy, may be used. When chemotherapy is required, multiagent regimens such as cyclophosphamide, vincristine, prednisolone (COP) are often used.

Conversely, approximately 55% of gastric lymphomas are high-grade lesions, which can occur with or without a low-grade MALT component [22]. These lymphomas are treated with chemotherapy and radiation therapy according to the extent of disease. In these aggressive lesions the cyclophosphamide, doxorubicin, vincristine, and prednisolone (CHOP) regimen has been the treatment most frequently employed. More recently rituximab, an anti-CD20 monoclonal antibody, has been either added to standard therapy or used alone, with encouraging results [31].

Surgical resection, once thought to be paramount in the diagnosis, staging, and treatment of early stage disease, is now used only in patients who develop complications of bleeding or perforation. In the German Multicenter Study group trial [22], 185 patients who had Stage I or II gastric lymphoma were enrolled, and treated with either gastrectomy followed by radiation, or chemotherapy plus radiation in the cases of high-grade lesions; versus chemotherapy and radiotherapy alone. In this nonrandomized trial, there was no significant difference in survival between the 79 patients receiving surgery and the 106 patients receiving nonoperative therapy, with overall 5-year survival rates of 82% and 84%, respectively. In this study, no patient experienced perforation, and there was only one case of hemorrhage in a patient treated with chemotherapy alone. Similarly, in a single-institution, prospective, randomized trial of chemotherapy versus chemotherapy plus surgery for Stage I and II lymphoma [26], Aviles and coworkers [32] noted no instances of perforation and only three instances of gastrointestinal bleeding in the chemotherapy group, versus two bleeding episodes in the surgery plus chemotherapy group. Thus, the authors conclude that patients who have early-stage, high-grade gastric lymphomas are best treated with chemotherapy or radiation therapy. Only rarely will these patients require surgical intervention for complications encountered during therapy. Patients who have locally advanced (Stage III) or disseminated gastric lymphoma (Stage IV) are universally treated with chemotherapy, with or without radiation. Surgery is occasionally indicated in such patients for residual disease confined to the stomach, or to palliate bleeding or obstruction that fails to resolve with nonoperative therapy. Primary surgical therapy is to be avoided in such cases because of the significant risk of complications and the delay in initiating systemic therapy.

Gastrointestinal stromal tumor

Although a relatively rare tumor, GIST is the most common sarcoma of the gastrointestinal tract [33]. The annual incidence is approximately 6000 cases in the United States alone, and the stomach is the most common site of involvement (60%–70%) [34]. The remainder occur in the small intestine (25%), rectum (5%), esophagus (2%), and a variety of other locations. Due to their appearance by light microscopy, GISTs were previously thought to be of smooth muscle origin, and the majority were classified as leiomyosarcomas [35]. Thus, extended gastric resection, often including contiguous organs, was advised. Recurrence after R0 resection occurred in approximately 50% of cases [36]. With the advent of immunohistochemistry and electron microscopy, it has become clear that these cells have both smooth muscle and neural elements, and the cell of origin is felt to be the interstitial cell of Cajal, an intestinal pacemaker cell [37]. In fact, the diagnosis of GIST is now secured by immunohistochemical staining for the tyrosine kinase receptor KIT (CD 117), which highlights the presence of interstitial cells of Cajal. Over 95% of GISTs exhibit unequivocal staining for KIT [34]. Approximately two thirds of GISTs will also express CD34. Histologically, these tumors exhibit a spindle-cell pattern, an epitheliod pattern or a mixed subtype.

The median age of incidence is 63 years, and tumors range between 0.5 and 44 cm at the time of diagnosis, with a median diameter of 6 cm [34]. Thus, these tumors may present with mass-related symptoms, such as abdominal pain, bloating, or early satiety. Another common presentation is melena or anemia due to overlying mucosal ulceration. A small subset of patients present with peritonitis caused by tumor rupture, with subsequent hemorrhage. Finally, many of these tumors are discovered incidentally during surgery, abdominal imaging, or endoscopy.

Although the majority of gastric GISTs will exhibit a benign course, there is a wide spectrum of biologic behavior. Among the prognostic factors examined, tumor size and mitotic rate appear to be the most valuable. Tumors less than 2 cm in size, with a mitotic count of less than five per high powered field (HPF) are considered to have a very low risk for an aggressive disease course. Conversely, tumors greater than 10 cm in size, or with greater than 10 mitoses per HPF, or greater than 5 cm with more than five mitoses per HPF are considered to be at high risk for aggressive clinical behavior. All others are considered to be of intermediate risk [34].

Patients who are suspected of having a GIST should undergo chest, abdominal, and pelvic imaging by either CT or MRI. Endoscopy with or without EUS may occasionally help with surgical planning, but rarely provides a tissue diagnosis because of infrequent mucosal involvement [38]. Surgical consultation should be obtained to determine whether the tumor is resectable. Biopsy is to be avoided in patients who have resectable tumors, because of the theoretical risk of tumor rupture with intra-abdominal dissemination. Biopsy may be required if the patient has widespread disease, or if entry on to a neoajuvant trial is being entertained. In these cases, biopsy may be obtained percutaneously, or at the time of EUS.

As opposed to gastric adenocarcinoma, the role of surgery in GIST is to resect the tumor with grossly negative margins, and an intact pseudocapsule. Because lymph node involvement is rare in GIST, no effort is made to perform an extended lymph node dissection. The tumor should be handled with care to avoid intra-abdominal rupture. Formal gastric resection is rarely required, and usually only indicated for lesions in close proximity to the pylorus or gastroesophageal junction (Fig. 1).

If the tumor is determined to be metastatic, or so locally advanced as to render surgical therapy excessively morbid, then patients are treated with

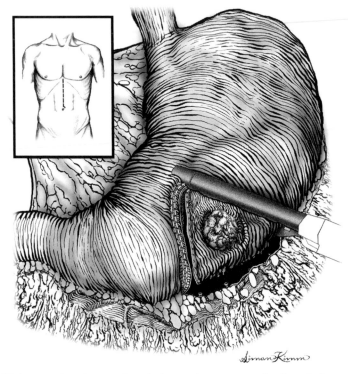

Fig. 1. Wedge resection of a gastrointestinal stromal tumor emanating from the lesser curve of the stomach.

the tyrosine kinase inhibitor imatinib mesylate. Imatinib is a selective inhibitor of a family of protein kinases, including the KIT-receptor tyrosine kinase (CD117), which is expressed in the majority of GISTs. Originally indicated for the treatment of chronic myelogenous leukemia, imatinib was approved for the treatment of KIT-positive GIST in 2002. Phase II clinical trials demonstrate a sustained objective response in a majority of patients who have advanced unresectable or metastatic GIST [39]. Patients who have borderline lesions should be treated until maximal response by CT and positron emission tomography (PET), and then surgery may be undertaken to resect and residual foci of disease. Similarly, although patients who have metastatic disease are unlikely to achieve a complete response to imatinib therapy, they should be periodically re-evaluated and considered for resection should this become technically feasible [38].

After a R0 resection of a GIST, no adjuvant therapy is indicated outside of a clinical trial. The American College of Surgeons Oncology Group (ACoSOG) is currently conducting two trials of imatinib in the postoperative setting. A Phase II trial (Z9000) of imatinib 400 mg/day for patients who have high-risk GIST, has reached accrual, and a Phase III trial randomizing patients who have intermediate risk GIST to 1 year of 400 mg/day of imatinib versus placebo (Z9001) is under way.

Gastric carcinoid

Gastric carcinoid tumors are rare, accounting for between 11% and 30% of all gastrointestinal neuroendocrine tumors, and fewer than 1% of all gastric tumors [40]. The median age at diagnosis is 62, and tumors are equally distributed among men and women. These lesions are often discovered during endoscopic evaluation for chronic abdominal pain. Other presenting symptoms include vomiting and diarrhea. These tumors rarely present with symptoms of the carcinoid syndrome. Diagnosis is usually confirmed by endoscopic biopsy, and EUS is helpful in determining the extent of gastric wall penetration and regional lymph node involvement.

Based primarily on their association with hypergastrinemia, gastric carcinoid tumors have been divided into three types. Type I tumors are associated with chronic atrophic gastritis, are generally small (<1 cm), and are often multiple and polypoid. Biologically, these lesions exhibit slow growth and only rarely metastasize to regional nodal basis or distant sites. Type II gastric carcinoid tumors are associated with the Zollinger-Ellison syndrome and multiple endocrine neoplasia (MEN)-Type I. These lesions are also usually small and multiple. Although they also grow at a slow rate, they may metastasize more frequently than Type I gastric carcinoids. The most biologically aggressive tumors are the Type III or sporadic gastric carcinoid tumors. These lesions are often large (>1 cm) at the time of diagnosis, and are not associated with hypergastrinemia. Type III lesions often exhibit metastasis to regional nodes (54%) and to the liver (24%) [40].

Endoscopic polypectomy or open resection via gastrotomy (local excision) is recommended in patients who have small, solitary Type I tumors. In the cases of multiple tumors or tumor recurrence, antrectomy is indicated to remove the source of hypergastrinemia. Patients who have Zollinger-Ellison or MEN-1 syndrome may be treated in a similar fashion to patients who have Type I lesions, with the extent of gastric resection being determined by the size and number of lesions. In contradistinction, patients who have Type III (sporadic) lesions require either distal or total gastrectomy with extended lymph node dissection [41]. All patients undergoing less than total gastrectomy should be followed by serial endoscopy at regular intervals [42].

Summary

Until recently, adjuvant therapy for gastric cancer was of little proven benefit. Thus, surgery was considered the sole mode of treatment for curative intent. This led many authors, especially in Asia, to propose radical, multivisceral resection with regional nodal dissection as a method for improving the dismal survival rates seen for patients who have adenocarcinoma of the stomach. Unfortunately, the benefit of extended gastric resection, either by total gastrectomy or with an extended D2 lymph node dissection, has never proven to be of benefit in terms of overall survival in a prospective, randomized trial from a Western center. Thus, it is the authors' current practice to perform a subtotal gastrectomy for antral lesions when a proximal margin of 5 to 6 cm can be obtained, and to perform dissection of all perigastric lymph nodes along the branches of the celiac axis. This will usually provide for the requisite 15 lymph nodes to be sampled for accurate staging, according to the 6th edition of the American Joint Committee on Cancer (AJCC) staging system.

General surgeons, gastrointestinal surgeons, and surgical oncologists alike will encounter less common gastric tumors such as gastric lymphoma, gastrointestinal stromal tumors, and gastric carcinoid tumors. Such tumors are often amenable to local resection, either by laparoscopic or open means, or may be treated by nonoperative means. Thus, techniques for limited gastric resection should be in the armamentarium of all such surgeons.

Finally, when faced with an unresectable tumor, it is now clear that operative intervention should be avoided to allow for early intervention with palliative or even potentially curative systemic therapy. This is true of GISTs, Stage IV adenocarcinoma, and Stage II and IV gastric lymphoma. Although palliative gastrectomy may be performed for intractable bleeding or perforation, it is almost always at the cost of a high rate of morbidity and postoperative mortality.

References

[1] Jamal A, Tiwari RC, Murray T, et al. Cancer statistics, 2004. CA Cancer J Clin 2004;54: 8–29.
[2] Cancer Statistics Working Group. United States cancer statistics: 1999–2001. Web-based incidence and mortality reports. Atlanta (GA): Department of Health and Human Services, Centers for Disease Control and Prevention, and National Cancer Institute; 2004. Available at: www.cdc.gov/cancer/npcr/uscs. Accessed April 3, 2005.
[3] Siewert JR, Bottcher K, Stein HJ, et al. Relevant prognostic factors in gastric cancer: ten-year results of the German Gastric Cancer Study. Ann Surg 1998;228(4):449–61.
[4] Hallissey MT, Jewkes AJ, Dunn JA, et al. Resection-line involvement in gastric cancer: a continuing problem. Br J Surg 1993;80(11):1418–20.
[5] Jakl RJ, Miholic J, Koller R, et al. Prognostic factors in adenocarcinoma of the cardia. Am J Surg 1995;169(3):316–9.
[6] Kooby DA, Coit DG. Controversies in the surgical management of gastric cancer. J of the National Comprehensive Cancer Network 2003;1(1):115–24.
[7] Gouzi JL, Huguier M, Fagniez PL, et al. Total versus subtotal gastrectomy for adeno-carcinoma of the gastric antrum. A French prospective controlled study. Ann Surg 1989; 209(2):162–6.

[8] Robertson CS, Chung SC, Woods SD, et al. A prospective randomized trial comparing R1 subtotal gastrectomy with R3 total gastrectomy for antral cancer. Ann Surg 1994;220(2): 176–82.

[9] Bozzetti F, Marubini E, Bonfanti G, et al. Subtotal versus total gastrectomy for gastric cancer: five-year survival rates in a multicenter randomized Italian trial. Italian Gastrointestinal Tumor Study Group. Ann Surg 1999;230(2):170–8.

[10] Spechler SJ. The role of gastric carditis in metaplasia and neoplasia at the gastroesophageal junction. Gastroenterology 1999;117(1):218–28.

[11] Devesa SS, Blot WJ, Fraumeni JF Jr. Changing patterns in the incidence of esophageal and gastric carcinoma in the United States. Cancer 1998;83(10):2049–53.

[12] Rudiger Siewert J, Feith M, Werner M, et al. Adenocarcinoma of the esophagogastric junction: results of surgical therapy based on anatomical/topographic classification in 1002 consecutive patients. Ann Surg 2000;232(3):353–61.

[13] Harrison LE, Karpeh MS, Brennan MF. Total gastrectomy is not necessary for proximal gastric cancer. Surgery 1998;123(2):127–30.

[14] Miner TJ, Jaques DP, Karpeh MS, et al. Defining palliative surgery in patients receiving noncurative resections for gastric cancer. J Am Coll Surg 2004;198(6):1013–21.

[15] ReMine WH. Palliative operations for incurable gastric cancer. World J Surg 1979;3(6): 721–9.

[16] Monson JR, Donohue JH, McIlrath DC, et al. Total gastrectomy for advanced cancer. A worthwhile palliative procedure. Cancer 1991;68(9):1863–8.

[17] Hartgrink HH, Putter H, Klein Kranenbarg E, et al. Dutch Gastric Cancer Group. Value of palliative resection in gastric cancer. Br J Surg 2002;89(11):1438–43.

[18] Nash CL, Gerdes H. Methods of palliation of esophageal and gastric cancer. Surg Oncol Clin N Am 2002;11(2):459–83.

[19] Adler DG, Baron TH. Endoscopic palliation of malignant gastric outlet obstruction using self-expanding metal stents: experience in 36 patients. Am J Gastroenterol 2002;97(1):72–8.

[20] Pyrhonen S, Kuitunen T, Nyandoto P, et al. Randomised comparison of fluorouracil, epidoxorubicin and methotrexate (FEMTX) plus supportive care with supportive care alone in patients with non-resectable gastric cancer. Br J Cancer 1995;71(3):587–91.

[21] Gurney KA, Cartwright RA, Gilman EA. Descriptive epidemiology of gastrointestinal non-Hodgkin's lymphoma in a population-based registry. Br J Cancer 1999;79(11–12):1929–34.

[22] Koch P, del Valle F, Berdel WE, et al. German Multicenter Study Group. Primary gastrointestinal non-Hodgkin's lymphoma: II. Combined surgical and conservative or conservative management only in localized gastric lymphoma—results of the prospective German Multicenter Study GIT NHL 01/92. J Clin Oncol 2001;19(18):3874–83.

[23] Crump M, Gospodarowicz M, Shepherd FA. Lymphoma of the gastrointestinal tract. Semin Oncol 1999;26(3):324–37.

[24] Non-Hodgkin's lymphoma, practice guidelines in oncology, v.1.2005. National Comprehensive Cancer Center Network. Available at: http://www.nccn.org/professionals/physician_gls/PDF/nhl.pdf. Accessed April 3, 2005.

[25] Talamonti MS. Gastric cancer. In: Winchester DP, Jones RS, Murphy GP, editors. Cancer surgery for the general surgeon. Philadelphia: Lippincott, Williams and Wilkins; 1998. p. 173–94.

[26] Yoon SS, Coit DG, Portlock CS, et al. The diminishing role of surgery in the treatment of gastric lymphoma. Ann Surg 2004;240(1):28–37.

[27] Parsonnet J, Hansen S, Rodriguez L, et al. *Helicobacter pylori* infection and gastric lymphoma. N Engl J Med 1994;330(18):1267–71.

[28] Isaacson PG. Recent developments in our understanding of gastric lymphomas. Am J Surg Pathol 1996;20(Suppl 1):S1–7.

[29] Stolte M, Bayerdorffer E, Morgner A, et al. *Helicobacter* and gastric MALT lymphoma. Gut 2002;50(Suppl 3):III19–24.

[30] Schechter NR, Yahalom J. Low-grade MALT lymphoma of the stomach: a review of treatment options. Int J Radiat Oncol Biol Phys 2000;46(5):1093–103.

[31] Martinelli G, Laszlo D, Ferreri AJ, et al. Clinical activity of rituximab in gastric marginal zone non-Hodgkin's lymphoma resistant to or not eligible for anti-*Helicobacter pylori* therapy. J Clin Oncol 2005;23(9):1979–83.

[32] Aviles A, Diaz-Maquoe JC, de la Torre A, et al. Is surgery necessary in the treatment of primary gastric non-Hodgkin lymphoma. Leuk Lymphoma 1991;5:365–9.

[33] Nilsson B, Bumming P, Meis-Kindblom JM, et al. Gastrointestinal stromal tumors: the incidence, prevalence, clinical course, and prognostication in the preimatinib mesylate era—a population-based study in western Sweden. Cancer 2005;103(4):821–9.

[34] Miettinen M, Sobin LH, Lasota J. Gastrointestinal stromal tumors of the stomach: a clinicopathologic, immunohistochemical, and molecular genetic study of 1765 cases with long-term follow-up. Am J Surg Pathol 2005;29(1):52–68.

[35] Ng EH, Pollock RE, Munsell MF, et al. Prognostic factors influencing survival in gastrointestinal leiomyosarcomas. Implications for surgical management and staging. Ann Surg 1992;215(1):68–77.

[36] Conlon KC, Casper ES, Brennan MF. Primary gastrointestinal sarcomas: analysis of prognostic variables. Ann Surg Oncol 1995;2(1):26–31.

[37] Corless CL, Fletcher JA, Heinrich MC. Biology of gastrointestinal stromal tumors. J Clin Oncol 2004;22(18):3813–25.

[38] Soft tissue sarcoma, practice guidelines in oncology, v.1.2005. National Comprehensive Cancer Center Network. Available at: www.nccn.org/professionals/physician_gls/PDF/sarcoma.pdf. Accessed April 3, 2005.

[39] Demetri GD, von Mehren M, Blanke CD, et al. Efficacy and safety of imatinib mesylate in advanced gastrointestinal stromal tumors. N Engl J Med 2002;347(7):472–80.

[40] Gilligan CJ, Lawton GP, Tang LH, et al. Gastric carcinoid tumors: the biology and therapy of an enigmatic and controversial lesion. Am J Gastroenterol 1995;90(3):338–52.

[41] Schindl M, Kaserer K, Niederle B. Treatment of gastric neuroendocrine tumors: the necessity of a type-adapted treatment. Arch Surg 2001;136(1):49–54.

[42] Modlin IM, Cornelius E, Lawton GP. Use of an isotopic somatostatin receptor probe to image gut endocrine tumors. Arch Surg 1995;130(4):367–73.

ELSEVIER
SAUNDERS

Surg Clin N Am 85 (2005) 1021–1032

SURGICAL
CLINICS OF
NORTH AMERICA

Radical Gastrectomy for Cancer of the Stomach

J. Lawrence Munson, MD*, Ruth O'Mahony, MD

Lahey Clinic Medical Center, 41 Mall Road, Burlington, MA 01805, USA

Cancer of the stomach was once the leading cause of cancer deaths in the United States, accounting for 38% of all cancer deaths in 1930 [1]. Since then, the incidence of stomach cancer has fallen in the United States (and the West in general), and now ranks as the fourteenth most common cancer in the United States [2]. This decrease in the West is not known to have been the result of planned public health measures or cancer screening efforts, but it does curiously correspond with evolution of better diet, decrease in smoking, increased vitamin C intake, and probable better, though inadvertent, control of *Helicobacter pylori* from extensive pediatric antibiotic use. Despite the decreasing incidence in the United States, over 20,000 people will be diagnosed yearly with stomach cancer, and over half will die from the disease [3]. The site of cancer has also changed, moving proximally to increased numbers of tumors of the cardia and gastroesophageal (GE) junction. In the last 2 decades, these proximal cancers have risen sharply, especially in patients younger than 40, from 10% to 30% of gastric cancers. This is most likely because the more distal tumors are those most likely to be affected by altering the risk factors. Despite the decreasing incidence of gastric cancer in the United States, the prognosis has remained stable for the last 2 decades: a dismal 10% to 20% 5-year survival. Adenocarcinoma accounts for 90% to 95% of gastric malignancies, with the rest being made up of sarcomas, lymphomas, and carcinoid tumors [1].

Lauren classification of stomach cancer

The Lauren classification (Table 1) recognizes two histologic types of gastric adenocarcinoma: intestinal and diffuse. The intestinal variety resembles typical colon cancers. Grossly, they may be nodular, polypoid

---

* Corresponding author.
E-mail address: John.L.Munson@lahey.org (J.L. Munson).

0039-6109/05/\$ - see front matter © 2005 Elsevier Inc. All rights reserved.
doi:10.1016/j.suc.2005.05.008   *surgical.theclinics.com*

Table 1
Lauren classification of stomach cancer

Intestinal	Diffuse
More common in endemic areas	More common in low prevalence areas
Associated with gastric atrophy	Associated with blood group A
Gland formation, intestinal metaplasia	Poorly differentiated, signet ring cells
Men > women	Women > men
Hematogenous spread	Lymphatic spread
Increasing incidence with age	Younger age group

or ulcerated, and they tend to be well demarcated. Histologically, the intestinal type has a well-formed glandular pattern. The diffuse type has a poorly defined border, with a plaquelike component, and is typically represented by linitis plastica. Microscopically, there are single cells, small groups, or cords of cells, with cytoplasmic mucin. The intestinal type of stomach cancer is most likely affected by environment and diet, and lends itself better to screening programs.

The predominant type of gastric adenocarcinoma in populations at highest risk is the intestinal type according to the Lauren his tological classification (see Table 1). In areas of the world where the incidence of gastric cancer is nearly epidemic, the histological type is most commonly the intestinal type. In Japan, the incidence is 70 per 100,000 men, and in the Andes region of South America, the incidence may reach 150 per 100,000, 20 times the incidence in the United States. The diffuse type is more prevalent in lower-risk populations.

The risk factors for gastric cancer in the United States are listed in Box 1.

Box 1. US gastric cancer risk factors [2]

- *H pylori* gastric infection
- Advanced age
- Male gender
- Diet low in fruit and vegetables
- Diets high in salted, smoked, or preserved foods
- Atrophic gastritis
- Gastric intestinal metaplasia
- Pernicious anemia
- Gastric adenomatous polyps
- Family history of gastric cancer
- Cigarette smoking
- Giant hypertrophic gastritis
- Familial adenomatous polyposis

Diagnosis of gastric cancer

Carcinoma of the stomach is much more likely to be diagnosed early in Japan, where 50% of cancers are considered "early gastric cancer." In the United States, only 10% to 15% are diagnosed early. The main reason for this is the aggressive screening program in Japan, relying on double-contrast upper gastrointestinal (GI) series and upper endoscopy with washings for cytology, and endoscopic biopsy. High-risk groups in this country, as identified in Box 1 above, should undergo routine surveillance endoscopy.

Most patients present late in the course of gastric cancer, and often with such nonspecific complaints as abdominal pain, weight loss, early satiety, nausea, reflux, and indigestion. When cancer has progressed to obstructing the stomach lumen, patients may exhibit progressive intolerance to foods, vomiting, and steady pain. Fatigue from malnutrition and anemia are usually very late signs. Because stomach cancer can spread via lymphatics, blood vessels, or by direct extension, physical findings can be varied as well. Lymphatic spread may be found in the left supraclavicular fossa, the Virchows' node. Hematogenous spread to the liver may manifest as a palpably enlarged liver or jaundice. Direct extension may reveal a mass in the epigastrium with relative fixation, or even transverse colon obstruction. Drop metastases may reveal themselves with a mass at the umbilicus (Sister Mary Joseph nodule), the pelvic floor (Blumer's shelf), or the ovary (Krukenburg tumor) [4].

Laboratory investigations should include complete cell counts, metabolic profile, liver chemistries, and tumor markers such as carcinoembryonic antigen (CEA) and carbohydrate antigen (CA) 19-9. These will help determine anemia, the relative amount of gastric outlet obstruction, and the possibility of liver metastases. CEA and CA 19-9 levels correlate with depth of tumor invasion, presence of lymphatic metastases, extent of tumor stage, and ultimately with patient survival [5].

Upper endoscopy is the best overall test to diagnose gastric cancer and determine location in the stomach. The addition of endoscopic ultrasound can help establish tumor (T) stage with an accuracy of about 73%. Helical CT scanning, especially when focused on the stomach, can help predict lymph node metastases [6,7].

The use of sentinel lymph-node biopsy to stage gastric cancer is still in its infancy, but there is reason to hope that it will be as useful as breast cancer sentinel-node biopsy. Two studies from South Korea [8,9] demonstrated that sentinel nodes could be accurately identified and harvested using 99mTc tin colloid peritumoral injection at the time of gastrectomy. There were no skip metastases found, and for lesions that were preoperatively determined to be stage T1 or T2, the sensitivity was 84% and the specificity was 100%. These patients would have been well-served with minimal lymphadenectomies.

Staging gastric carcinoma

Tumor, node, metasteses (TNM) staging used by the West is ultimately based on the histology of the resected specimen. The system from the American Joint Committee on Cancer (AJCC) is explained in the *AJCC Cancer Staging Handbook* [1]. The classification system used by the Japanese Research Society for Gastric Cancer differs from the American TNM system in the determination of nodal metastases.

In the Japanese system, node (N)1 is the invasion of perigastric nodes within 3 cm of the primary tumor, and N2 is invasion of nodes more than 3 cm from the tumor. In addition, the Japanese use N3 to denote retropancreatic, hepatoduodenal, portal, and mesenteric nodes. N4 is used to describe para-aortic and mesocolic nodes. The AJCC considers these N3 and N4 nodes to be distant metastases. The Japanese system uses lymph node stations rather than absolute number of nodes positive. Herein lies one of the controversies between the philosophies of gastric cancer staging and management: does the region of lymph nodes resected play a role in cure or just change the format of staging? As confusing as the staging systems can be, the definition of the resective therapies can be worse. Regardless of the confusion regarding staging, nomenclature, or definition of resections, surgical resection of stomach cancer offers the best prognosis for long-term survival, and the only chance for cure.

Surgical therapy of gastric cancer

The surgery for gastric cancer began in the nineteenth century when Theodor Bilroth first successfully resected an adenocarcinoma of the antrum with a distal gastrectomy. Although not the first to attempt resection, Bilroth had the first survivor, with the patient dying 4 months later of disseminated disease [10]. For the next half century, advances in both anesthesia and surgery encouraged the extension of gastric surgery to more radical resections. Bilroth's "pylorectomy" resection gave way to radical total gastrectomy as treatment of choice by the 1940s [11]. Over the next several decades, controversy over whether the added morbidity and mortality of total gastrectomy over subtotal gastrectomy was accompanied by any improved survival persuaded most surgeons to use radical subtotal excisions for all but proximal cancers. The only hope for cure of stomach cancer in 2005 remains complete surgical extirpation of the cancer with an adequate margin of normal tissue. The Lauren classification of the primary tumor predicts the likelihood of intramural spread, and thus determines what is considered an adequate resection margin. For the intestinal type tumors, 3 cm of margin is considered adequate, whereas for the diffuse type, 5 cm of margin is required [12]. Distally, resection of 2 cm of uninvolved duodenum is adequate. Some authors have suggested that because gastric cancers characteristically have extensive intramural spread, the resection margins should be at least 6 cm to ensure microscopically negative margins and a low rate of anastomotic recurrence [13]. As the histological type of the tumor is not usually known at the time of surgery, the authors feel it reasonable to strive for a 5 to 6 cm proximal margin. The addition of en-bloc removal of affected organs, such as the spleen, pancreas, colon, and lateral segment of the left lobe of the liver (Segments II and III), is considered appropriate for contiguous spread of the primary as long as no dissemination of the primary is apparent. Recent work from Memorial Sloan-Kettering Cancer Center in New York city demonstrates equivalent mortality for gastric resection with and without en-bloc resection of adjacent organs [14]; however, the morbidity rates were higher in the group requiring splenectomy and distal pancreatectomy. More postoperative interventions were also necessary to treat complications in this group. Other retrospective reviews and randomized controlled trials have demonstrated increased morbidity and mortality from splenopancreatectomy [15].

The major controversy regarding therapy now is in regard to the extent of lymph node dissection necessary to accomplish realistic expectation of cure versus the frequent reality of palliation that are not explained by environment or genetics. No doubt that some of the confusion arises from differences in patient populations between the United States and Japan, beyond environmental and genetic differences. As stated above, in Japan, 50% of patients are diagnosed with early gastric cancer, but fewer than 15% of United States' patients are found this early [1]. Early gastric cancer, not to be confused with carcinoma in situ, refers to cancers that are restricted to the mucosa and submucosa, without regard for nodal status [16].

The behavior and beliefs of surgeons around the world have swung through broad arcs as studies from the East and West have tried to provide justification for more or less radical resections, and their associated lymph node dissections. There are two types of resection for the purposes of this discussion: radical total, or radical subtotal resections of the stomach. The terminology becomes confusing when one looks at the literature defining resections and defining the lymph node areas for removal and staging. Earlier studies define R1 resections as being complete tumor removal, along with removal of the first tier of perigastric lymph nodes. The perigastric nodes are left and right pericardial, the lesser curvature, the greater curvature, the suprapyloric, and the infrapyloric nodes. R2 resections were considered those that removed the entire tumor, the first tier of lymph nodes, and the second tier of extraperigastric nodes—those located along the vascular supply of the stomach. This second tier is comprised of the nodes along the left gastric artery, the common hepatic artery, the celiac axis, the splenic hilum, the splenic artery, the hepatoduodenal ligament, the root of the mesentery, the middle colic artery, retropancreatic nodes, and the para-aortic nodes. This classification came out of the Japanese Research Society for Gastric Cancer based upon work by Maruyama and colleagues [17].

Confusion arises when looking at Western data based on the AJCC TNM system, which considers an R0 resection to mean a histologically proven complete tumor excision, an R1 excision meaning one with residual microscopic tumor (positive margins), and an R2 excision meaning one with residual macroscopic tumor (tumor transected). Current literature considers the previous Japanese R1 resections as D1, the R2 as D2, and even more extensive resections to include distant nodal fields as D3 and D4 resections (Figs. 1–3). There are also differences in staging by nodal status on final pathology. Some literature is based on the Japanese N1 and N2 stations as positive nodes in the perigastric or extraperigastric respectively, versus the AJCC system that counts N1 and N2 by absolute number of positive nodes, irrespective of their location in the resected specimen (Figs. 4, 5).

There are considerable differences in the actual prosection of gastrectomy specimens, because the absolute number of nodes found differs significantly between Eastern and Western analyses. More lymph nodes are typically analyzed in Japanese specimens compared with American prosections, with an average of 62 per specimen in Japan versus 12 at Memorial Sloan-Kettering [18]. Does more careful or meticulous lymphadenectomy result in more accurate staging of cancer in Japan [18,19]? The Japanese have most precisely described the lymphatic stations for gastric cancer [20], as seen in Fig. 4. Lymph node basins are numbered and then grouped based upon the location of the primary tumor. A D1 lymphadenectomy refers to removal of group 1 lymph nodes. A D2 lymphadenectomy denotes removal of group 1 and group 2 nodes (see Figs. 1–3). D3 dissection includes group 1, 2, and 3 nodes. D4 dissection includes group 1, 2, 3, and para-aortic nodes.

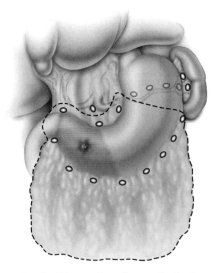

Fig. 1. Extent of resection for D1 resection of tumor in distal one third of stomach.

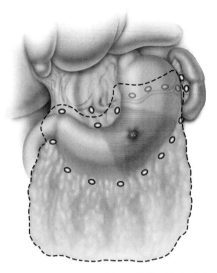

Fig. 2. D1 resection for tumors of the middle third of the stomach.

What is the evidence that extent of resection and extent of lymph node excision can impact overall survival? D1 lymphadenectomy is routinely performed in the United States, whereas D2 lymphadenectomy is routinely practiced in Japan. Survival benefit with D2 dissection was first demonstrated in Japan in 1981. Kodama and coworkers [21] found that 5-year survival with D2 dissection was 39%, versus 18% with D1 resection.

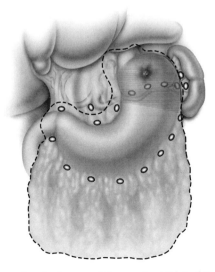

Fig. 3. D1 resection for tumors of the proximal third of the stomach.

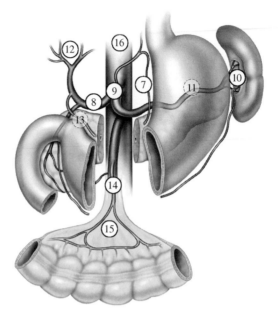

Fig. 4. Extraperigastric nodes: (7) left gastric artery; (8) common hepatic artery; (9) celiac artery; (10) splenic hilum; (11) splenic artery; (12) hepatic pedicle; (13) retropancreatic; (14) mesenteric root; (15) middle colic artery; (16) para-aortic.

Other groups in Japan also seemed to demonstrate this effect, and even went on to routinely advocate splenectomy and distal pancreatectomy to ensure complete excision of nodal stations 10 and 11 [22]. Further trials, however, demonstrated greatly increased morbidity associated with routine pancreatosplenectomy [22,23]. For this and other reasons, the authors do not

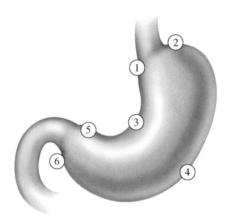

Fig. 5. Perigastric nodes: (1) right pericardial; (2) left pericardial; (3) lesser curvature; (4) greater curvature; (5) suprapyloric; (6) infrapyloric.

recommend removal of the spleen and pancreas solely for the purpose of lymph node clearance.

German studies [24] have shown that there may be a benefit to aggressive lymphadenectomy in patients who have Stage II or IIIa tumors; however, they suggest that the ratio of positive nodes to negative nodes resected may be an independent prognostic index. They also suggest that 5-year survival can double if more than 25 nodes are resected. The use of ratios in this manner simply inserts bias into the data to suggest that more nodes need to be resected. As Cady [25] has well explained, resecting more lymph nodes does not alter survival, so resecting more negative nodes certainly will not.

Western trials have not duplicated the benefit of D2 dissections that the Japanese trials are believed to have shown. A British trial [26] demonstrated significantly higher morbidity (28% for D1 versus 46% for D2) and mortality (6.5% for D1 versus 13% for D2) for D2 lymphadenectomy, with no difference in 5-year survival. A Dutch trial [27] also showed almost double the morbidity and mortality for D2 versus D1 dissections, with no survival benefit conferred by extended lymphadenectomy. A number of theories have attempted to explain the disparity in results between Japan and the West. Because of the meticulous labeling and dissection techniques used in Japan, it has been suggested that more accurate staging occurs [18,19]. This implies that Western specimens are understaged and cannot be compared well to Japanese specimens. There is also the possibility that gastric cancer is a less aggressive, biologically different disease in the Japanese population. Review of data from the National Cancer Database [28] demonstrates higher survival rates for Japanese-Americans than for Americans of European descent. Additionally, Japanese-Americans had a lower incidence of T4 disease, supporting the idea that gastric cancer in Japanese is a less virulent disease. Furthermore, as stated above, population-based screening initiatives in Japan lead to detection of more gastric cancers at earlier stages [29]. It seems, therefore, reasonable to suggest that the survival benefit in Japan is due to factors other than just more aggressive surgical resection.

Lastly, there is now an increasingly popular theory in Japan that is advocating minimal surgery, even mucosectomy alone, for early gastric cancer. Studies are showing excellent survival despite abandoning the D2 standard resection. This also seems to imply a difference in tumor biology in the Asian population [30].

General preoperative recommendations

All patients are staged with endoscopy, helical CT scan, chest x-ray, comprehensive metabolic profile, complete blood count, and tumor markers CEA and CA19-9. Tumors that are proximal, cardia, or GE junction are additionally studied with endoscopic ultrasound (EUS). A bowel prep is administered the day before surgery should colon resection be necessary. In addition, if splenectomy and distal pancreatectomy are anticipated, immunizations for the asplenic state are given. The authors recommend the use of epidural anesthesia for postoperative pain control.

Surgical resection based upon tumor location

Tumors of the proximal third of the stomach account for about 30% of all gastric cancers in the West. These are different from tumors of the GE junction, which are usually treated as esophageal cancers. For proximal gastric cancers, surgeons are fairly split between esophagogastrectomy via a combined upper midline and right thoracotomy (Ivor-Lewis), and radical total gastrectomy. Although the two procedures may be equivalent for tumor removal, proximal gastric resection is associated with higher rates of reflux esophagitis and dumping than total gastrectomy [31]. Additionally, the Norwegian Stomach Cancer Trial [32] demonstrated mortality rates for proximal gastric resection that were double those for total gastrectomy. When performing total gastrectomy for proximal cancer, the authors strive for an esophageal margin of 6 cm. Lymph node dissection should be D1 (perigastric), and should include left and right cardia nodes, short gastric nodes, and nodes along both greater and lesser curves. Reconstruction should be with Roux-en-Y esophagojejunostomy.

Tumors of the middle third of the stomach can be treated with either total gastrectomy, or near-total gastrectomy if a 5 to 6 cm margin is possible. If a near-total gastrectomy is done, care must be exercised to leave an adequate blood supply to the cuff of remnant gastric tissue to allow a safe anastomosis. Nodal dissection should be perigastric, D1, and should include nodes along the greater and lesser curves, short gastric, and infra- and suprapyloric areas. Reconstruction is also by means of Roux-en-Y.

Tumors of the distal third of the stomach are generally treated with radical subtotal gastrectomy. This implies a proximal resection line about the level of the descending branch of the left gastric artery, if a 5 to 6 cm margin can be obtained. Distally, the authors look for 2 cm of normal duodenum. Lymph node dissection is again D1, and includes those nodes along both curvatures, as well as supra- and infrapyloric areas. Reconstruction is by antecolic Bilroth II, or Roux-en-Y gastrojejunostomy. Bilroth I reconstructions are generally not done for cancer; however, early gastric cancer can sometimes be managed safely in this manner, provided adequate margins are obtained.

Summary

Although there has been progress in the treatment of gastric cancer, the overall prognosis for these patients remains grim. Chemotherapy and radiation have not convincingly demonstrated neoadjuvant benefit.

Consequently, surgical resection remains the mainstay of treatment. Although some patients in Japan may be seen as candidates for endoscopic or wedge resection of early mucosal cancers, this represents a very small percentage of gastric cancers, particularly in the West. Most patients require a radical resection, to include the primary tumor, 5 to 6 cm of normal tissue around the tumor, the perigastric nodes, and the greater omentum. Lymphadenectomy beyond the D1 level has not been shown to confer a survival advantage in the West. For this reason, it is not recommended unless grossly positive nodes are present within a particular nodal basin. Resection of additional organs, such as distal pancreas or spleen, can add significantly to the morbidity of the operation, and should therefore be limited to those patients who have direct tumor invasion of these structures.

References

[1] Stomach. In: Greene F, Page P, Fleming I, et al, editors. AJCC cancer staging handbook. 6th edition. New York: Springer Verlag; 2002. p. 99–103.
[2] Gastric cancer (PDQ) treatment. National Cancer Institute, 2/12/2004.
[3] Godellas CV. Gastric cancer. In: Sacclarides, Millikan, Godellas CV, editors. Surgical oncology, an algorithmic approach. New York: Springer-Verlag; 2003. p. 266–71.
[4] Patino JF. Gastric cancer. In: Cameron J, editor. Current surgical therapy. 6th edition. St. Louis (MO): Mosby; 1998. p. 108–14.
[5] Mihmanli M, Dilege E, Demir U, et al. The use of tumor markers as predictors of prognosis in gastric cancer. Hepatogastroenterology 2004;51(59):1544–7.
[6] Polkowski M, Palucki J, Wronska E, et al. Endosonography versus helical computed tomography for locoregional staging of gastric cancer. Endoscopy 2004;36(7):617–23.
[7] Haberman CR, Weiss F, Riecken R, et al. Preoperative staging of gastric adenocarcinoma: comparison of helical CT and endoscopic US. Radiology 2004;230:465–71.
[8] Kim MC, Jung GJ, Lee JH, et al. Sentinel lymph node biopsy with 99mTc tin colloid in patients with gastric carcinoma. Hepatogastroenterology 2003;50(Suppl 2):ccxiv–xv.
[9] Kim MC, Kim HH, Jung GJ, et al. Lymphatic mapping and sentinel node biopsy using 99mTc tin colloid in gastric cancer. Ann Surg 2004;239(3):383–7.
[10] Herrington JL. Gastric cancer. In: Cameron J, editor. Current surgical therapy. 5th edition. St. Louis (MO): Mosby; 1995. p. 89–93.
[11] Longmire W. Total gastrectomy for carcinoma of the stomach. Surg Gynecol Obstet 1947; 84:21–5.
[12] Sewart JR, Fink U, Sendler A, et al. Gatric Cancer. Curr Probl Surg 1997;34:835–942.
[13] Papachristou DN, Fortner JG. Local recurrence of gastric adenocarcinomas after gastrectomy. J Surg Oncol 1981;18:47–53.
[14] Martin RC 2nd, Jacques DP, Brennan MF, et al. Achieving R0 resection for locally advanced gastric cancer: is it worth the risk of multi-organ resection? J Am Coll Surg 2002; 194:568–77.
[15] Piso P, Bellin T, Aselmann H, et al. Results of combined gastrectomy and pancreatic resection in patients with advanced primary gastric carcinoma. Dig Surg 2002;19(4): 281–5.
[16] Farley DR, Donahue JH. Early gastric cancer. Surg Clin N Am 1992;72(2):401–22.
[17] Maruyama K, Gunven P, Okabayashi K, et al. Lymph node metastases of gastric cancer:general pattern in 1931 patients. Ann Surg 1989;210:596–602.
[18] Brennan MF. Radical surgery for gastric cancer. A review of the Japanese experience. Cancer 1989;64:2063.

[19] Bunt AMG, Hermans J, Smit VTHBM, et al. Surgical/pathologic-stage migration confounds comparison of gastric cancer survival rates between Japan and Western countries. J Clin Oncol 1995;13:19–25.

[20] Kajitani T. Japanese Research Society for the Study of Gastric Cancer: the general rules for gastric cancer study in surgery and pathology. Jpn J Surg 1981;11:127–45.

[21] Kodama Y, Sugimachi K, Soejima K, et al. Evaluation of extensive lymph node dissection for carcinoma of the stomach. World J Surg 1981;5:241–8.

[22] Kasakura Y, Fujii M, Mochizuki F, et al. Is there a benefit of pancreaticosplenectomy with gastrectomy for advanced gastric cancer? Am J Surg 2000;179:237–42.

[23] Cuschieri A, Fayers P, Fielding J, et al. Postoperative morbidity and mortality after D1 and D2 resections for gastric cancer: preliminary results of the MRC randomized controlled surgical trial. Surgical Cooperatve Group. Lancet 1996;347:995–9.

[24] Siewart JR, Bottcher K, Stein HJ, et al, and the German Gastric Carcinoma Study Group. Relevant prognostic factors in gastric cancer: 10-year results of the German Gastric Cancer Study. Ann Surg 1998;228:449–61.

[25] Cady B. Commentary on "Multidisciplinary approach to esophageal and gastric cancer" by Stein et al. Surg Clin N Am 2000;80:683–6.

[26] Cuschieri A, Weeden S, Fielding J, et al. Patient survival after D1 and D2 resections for gastric cancer: long-term results of the MRC randomized surgical trial. Surgical Cooperative Group. Br J Cancer 1999;79:1522–30.

[27] Bonenkamp JJ, Hermans J, Sasako M, et al. Extended lymph-node dissection for gastric cancer. Dutch Gastric Cancer Group. N Engl J Med 1999;340:908–14.

[28] Hundahl SA. The National Cancer Data Base report on poor survival of US gastric carcinoma patients treated with gastrectomy: 5th edition. American Joint Committee on Cancer staging, proximal disease, and the "different disease" hypothesis. Cancer 2000;88:921–32.

[29] Gervasoni JE, Taneja C, Chung MA, et al. Biological and clinical significance of lymphadenectomy. Surg Clin North Am 2000;80:1631–73.

[30] Theuer CP, Kurosaki T, Ziogas A, et al. Asian patients with gastric carcinoma in the United States exhibit unique clinical features and superior overall and cancer specific survival rates. Cancer 2000;89:1883–92.

[31] Buhl K, Schlag P, Herfarth C. Quality of life and functional results following different types of resection for gastric carcinoma. Eur J Surg Oncol 1990;16:404–9.

[32] Viste A, Haugstvedt T, Eide GE, et al. Postoperative complications and mortality after surgery for gastric cancer. Ann Surg 1988;207:7–13.

ELSEVIER
SAUNDERS

SURGICAL
CLINICS OF
NORTH AMERICA

Surg Clin N Am 85 (2005) 1033–1051

Adjuvant and Neoadjuvant Therapy for Gastric Cancer

Ricardo J. Gonzalez, MD,
Paul F. Mansfield, MD*

*Department of Surgical Oncology, The University of Texas MD Anderson Cancer Center,
Unit 444, 1515 Holcombe Boulevard, Houston, TX 77030-5235, USA*

The incidence of gastric cancer in the United States has declined since the 1930s, when gastric cancer was the leading cause of cancer-specific mortality in United States men [1]. According to the Surveillance, Epidemiology, and End Results (SEER) database [2], the age adjusted incidence for all races was 9.1 per 100,000 for 1992–2002. Gastric cancer is more common among men than women, and in the United States, African Americans, Hispanics, and Native Americans are 1.5 to 2.5 times more likely than whites to develop gastric cancer [3]. Although the incidence of gastric cancer is declining throughout the world, it is still the second-leading cause of cancer-specific mortality worldwide, one of the most common malignancies in China, South America, Eastern Europe, and Japan, and the leading cause of death in Korea [4,5].

Clinical manifestations

The symptoms of gastric cancer are often nonspecific, frequently leading to a delay in presentation and diagnosis at an advanced stage. The most common symptoms at diagnosis are abdominal pain (50%–65% of patients) and weight loss (40% of patients). Although anemia is a frequent finding, clinically significant and potentially life-threatening upper gastrointestinal bleeding is less common and occurs in only 10% to 17% of patients. The authors' analyses of over 1000 cases of gastric cancer seen at The University of Texas MD Anderson Cancer Center indicate that symptoms may vary by

* Corresponding author.
E-mail address: pmansfie@mdanderson.org (P.F. Mansfield).

0039-6109/05/$ - see front matter © 2005 Elsevier Inc. All rights reserved.
doi:10.1016/j.suc.2005.05.004
surgical.theclinics.com

the location of the primary lesion. Nausea and vomiting are more common among patients who have a nonproximal cancer (26%), whereas dysphagia occurs predominantly among patients who have proximal cancer localization (38%). Early satiety can be especially prominent among patients who have diffuse infiltration or linitis plastica.

Findings detectable on physical examination are late events that usually indicate advanced, unresectable disease. A palpable epigastric mass indicates a large, locally advanced tumor, and jaundice usually indicates hepatic metastasis or metastatic lymphadenopathy in the portal region. Drop metastasis to the pelvis can present as a Blumer's shelf, or ovarian metastasis can present as Krukenberg's tumor. A periumbilical mass can arise from lymph node metastasis or, more commonly, from peritoneal metastasis. Other sites of palpable lymphadenopathy are in the left supraclavicular area, Virchow's node, or in the left axilla. Other less common dermatological findings include acanthosis nigricans and multiple seborrheic keratoses.

Pattern of spread

Gastric cancer is a generally aggressive disease that can spread by several mechanisms. Adjacent organs such as the diaphragm, esophagus, liver, pancreas, spleen, and colon may be involved by direct extension. Spread can also occur through the rich network of gastric lymphatics to local and distant nodes. The hematogenous route can lead to hepatic involvement or, less commonly, to lung, bone, and brain metastasis. Finally, as the cancer penetrates the gastric wall, peritoneal metastasis and carcinomatosis frequently occur. Ovarian metastasis may develop in the absence of peritoneal carcinomatosis.

Organ failure due to liver and peritoneal metastases is a frequent cause of death. Japanese investigators have noted that histology and patient age might affect the pattern of gastric cancer metastases. In an autopsy study of 173 cases of gastric cancer [6], investigators found that a glandular histology was associated with hepatic metastases, and that a diffuse histology was associated with peritoneal metastases. Peritoneal metastases were also more common among younger patients. In a separate surgical study [7], the case records of 216 patients who had synchronous hepatic or peritoneal metastases were analyzed. Peritoneal metastases were associated with poorly differentiated or signet ring cell histology, whereas well- to moderately differentiated histology was more common among patients who had hepatic metastases.

The authors recently analyzed patterns of metastasis among 494 gastric cancer patients who had synchronous hepatic or peritoneal metastasis treated at MD Anderson Cancer Center [8]. In multivariate analyses, well- to moderately differentiated histology, proximal gastric cancer, male gender, and white race were more commonly associated with hepatic metastases. Peritoneal metastases were associated with mucinous or signet ring histology, nonproximal gastric cancer localization, female gender, and nonwhite race.

Adjuvant therapy

Although surgery remains the only proven curative option for localized gastric cancer, long-term survival rates after surgery alone remain sub-optimal for all but the earliest disease stage (T1 N0 M0); this is especially true in Western countries. A recent report by the National Cancer Database [9] showed the 5-year survival rates of American patients who had Stages Ib, II, IIIa, and IIIb gastric cancer to be 58%, 34%, 20%, and 8%, respectively. In an attempt to improve survival rates and reduce the rate of recurrence, researchers have designed trials investigating the potential utility of adjuvant and neoadjuvant therapy.

Adjuvant therapy is given after a potentially curative resection to reduce or eliminate the possibility of recurrence of cancer at local or distant sites, whereas neoadjuvant therapy is given before an anticipated definitive surgical procedure. Adjuvant or neoadjuvant therapy may include chemo-therapy (systemic or intraperitoneal), immunotherapy, radiotherapy, or any combination of these. Although definitive surgery is the best chance for cure, 5-year survival rates remain below 50% in the latest randomized trial [10], even after curative gastrectomy followed by postoperative chemoradio-therapy. Efforts to improve survival rates have led to numerous adjuvant and neoadjuvant (discussed later) therapy trials, starting in the mid 1970s.

Chemotherapy

Numerous trials have studied systemic chemotherapy in the adjuvant setting, often with disappointing results. Many of the early trials lacked adequate statistical power, included improper control groups, or had suboptimal methodologies. Their treatment regimens and inclusion criteria were heterogeneous, because accurate staging was not available. These limitations made some of their results nonreproducible [11]. Meta-analyses of these trials are fraught with difficulties, and a particular regimen cannot be recommended on the basis of such heterogeneous data. Nonetheless, two large analyses were performed, with conflicting results [12,13]. Each analysis recommended adjuvant chemotherapy for subgroups such as node-positive or Asian patients. Current chemotherapy regimens are likely of only marginal benefit for patients who have undergone curative resection, and adjuvant chemotherapy is not recommended outside of a clinical trial. A summary of chemotherapy trials for gastric cancer is included in Table 1 [14–30]. Because of the heterogeneity of these trials, only those reporting benefit are discussed below.

Table 1
Selected postoperative adjuvant therapy trials

Treatment groups	Stage	No. of patients	Survival rate (%)	P value	Reference
Chemotherapy					
MMC	I–IV	242	68 at 5 years	0.05	[14]
Surgery alone	R0	283	53 at 5 years		
MMC	T1 N1–2 or	68	41 at 5 years	<0.025	[15]
Surgery alone	T2–3 NX	66	26 at 5 years		
MeCCNU + 5-FU	T1–4 NX M0	71	NS	<0.03*	[16]
Surgery alone	with R0	71	NS		
MeCCNU + 5-FU	T1–4 NX	66	38 at 3.5 years	NS	[17]
Surgery alone	M0, R0	68	39 at 3.5 years		
MeCCNU + 5-FU	T1–4 NX M0	91	57 at 2 years	NS	[18]
Surgery alone		89	57 at 2 years		
FAM	I, II, III	93	37 at 5 years	NS	[19]
Surgery alone		100	32 at 5 years		
FAM	II, III	155	43 at 5 years	NS	[20]
Surgery alone		159	40 at 5 years		
FAM	Ib–IV	133	45 at 5 years	NS	[21]
Surgery alone		148	35 at 5 years		
FAM	II, III, IV	138	19 at 5 years	NS	[22]
Radiotherapy		153	12 at 5 years		
Surgery alone		145	20 at 5 years		
5-FU + doxorubicin	I, II, III, IV	61	32 at 5 years	NS	[23]
Surgery alone		64	33 at 5 years		
Epirubicin + folinic acid + 5-FU	T1–3 N1–2	55	25 at 3 years	<0.01	[24]
Surgery alone		48	13 at 3 years		
5-FU + MMC	II, III, IV, Include residual disease	141	11 at 5 years	NS	[25]
5-FU + MMC + CMFV course 1		140	17 at 5 years		
Surgery alone		130	12 at 5 years		
MMC	T1 N1–2,	45	44 at 5 years	0.04	[26]
MMC + tegafur	T2–3 NX	40	67 at 5 years		
MMC + UFT	II, III	69	NS	NS	[27]
Surgery alone		75	NS		
Chemoimmunotherapy					
5-FU + MeCCNU	T1–4 NX M0	75	50 at 5 years	NS	[28]
5-FU + MeCCNU + levamisole		69	50 at 5 years		
Surgery alone		69	50 at 5 years		
MFC	T1 N1–2 M0	NS	NS	NS	[29]
MFC + picibanil	T2–4 NX M0	NS	NS		
Surgery alone		NS	NS		
MMC + 5-FU + Ara-C + OK-432	III	74	45 at 5 years	<0.05	[30]
Surgery alone		64	23 at 5 years		

* Log rank testing revealed $P = 0.06$; covariate analysis showed $P < 0.03$.

Abbreviations: Ara-C, cytarabine; CMFV, cyclophosphamide, methotrexate, 5-fluorouracil, and vincristine; FAM, 5-fluorouracil, doxorubicin, and mitomycin C; 5-FU, 5-fluorouracil; MeCCNU, methyl-lomustine; MFC, mitomycin C, 5-fluorouracil, and cytarabine; MMC, mitomycin C; NS, not stated; R0, complete resection; UFT, uracil plus tegafur.

Most chemotherapy agents considered active in advanced gastric cancer have reported response rates of 15% to 20% as single agents. Thus, to detect the expected survival benefit, randomized trials involving hundreds to thousands of patients would be necessary. The activity of single-agent mito-mycin in the adjuvant setting was first reported by Japanese investi-gators in 1977 [14]. The investigators summarized four trials of adjuvant mitomycin, only one of which showed an improved 5-year survival rate in treated patients compared with controls (68% versus 53%; $P = .05$). A sub-sequent small trial from Spain [15] also reported a survival advantage for mitomycin compared with surgery (41% versus 26%; $P < 0.025$). The higher survival rates with single-agent mitomycin seen in two of these five trials must be balanced by the first trial's lack of reproducibility and the second trial's small number of patients. The many trials of mitomycin-containing regimens that have demonstrated no survival benefit must also be considered [19–22,25,27,31].

Higher response rates have been reported with combination chemother-apy than with single-agent regimens. Early postoperative combination chemotherapy trials used 5-fluorouracil (5-FU) and methyl-lomustine (MeCCNU). In one trial, the Gastrointestinal Tumor Study Group [16] randomized 142 patients to receive surgery alone or surgery followed by 2 years of adjuvant chemotherapy with 5-FU and MeCCNU. After a median follow-up of 4 years, a significant ($P < 0.03$) survival benefit was reported for patients treated with chemotherapy. The median survival duration was 33 months for the surgery-only arm and more than 4 years in the adjuvant chemotherapy arm. Subsequent randomized trials of these agents by the Veterans Administration Surgical Oncology Study Group [32] and the Eastern Cooperative Oncology Group [18] showed no survival advantage or reduction in risk of recurrence for this adjuvant chemotherapy regimen versus surgery alone.

More recently, investigators randomly assigned 103 patients to surgery followed by treatment with epirubicin, 5-FU, and folinic acid or surgery alone [24]. After a follow up period of 36 months, 21 (25%) treated patients and 7 (13%) control patients were alive ($P < 0.01$) The median survival duration was significantly greater for treated versus untreated patients (20.4 versus 13.6 months; $P < 0.05$); however, this was a small trial, with only 55 patients receiving treatment.

The use of an oral 5-FU pro-drug is an attractive approach. In one trial [26], 85 patients were randomly assigned to treatment with mitomycin every 6 weeks for four cycles or mitomycin at the same dosage with daily oral tegafur for 36 consecutive days each cycle. The 5-year survival rate was significantly better in the group receiving mitomycin and tegafur (67% versus 44%; $P = .04$), but the small number of patients, a long accrual time (11 years), and the lack of a control group suggest these data should be reviewed cautiously. Larger trials comparing similar oral fluoropyrimidines and mitomycin with surgery alone have yielded negative results [27,31].

Intraperitoneal therapy

The peritoneal cavity is a frequent site of relapse for patients who have gastric cancer. Delivery of chemotherapy through an intraperitoneal (IP) route theoretically could improve the treatment of microscopic residual disease. Several trials have examined the feasibility of such an approach. Initial work by Schiessel and colleagues [33] and Sautner and coworkers [34] compared surgery alone to surgery followed by intraperitoneal cisplatin. No survival differences were observed, but both trials included patients who had metastatic disease and thus were not true adjuvant therapy trials.

Japanese investigators used intraperitoneal carbon-adsorbed mitomycin in a study of 50 patients who had gastric cancer and serosal infiltration and who were randomly assigned to receive intraperitoneal treatment or surgery alone [35]. A significant 3-year survival rate advantage was observed for the 24 treated patients (69% versus 27%; $P < 0.01$); however, when Rosen and colleagues [36] attempted to confirm the advantage of this strategy in a larger Austrian trial, the trial was closed early because of increased postoperative morbidity and mortality in the treated group. Yu and coworkers [37] conducted a well-designed randomized study of combination intraperitoneal chemotherapy with mitomycin and 5-FU, the results of which were reassessed after prolonged follow-up. Investigators randomly assigned 248 patients to receive surgery alone or surgery and early postoperative intraperitoneal chemotherapy via internal catheters for the first 5 postoperative days. Patient characteristics and extent of surgical resection were similar in both groups. Although the incidence of mortality was not significantly different, the patients in the study group had a higher incidence of abscess formation (14% versus 4%; $P < 0.05$) and bleeding (10% versus 1%; $P < 0.05$). The overall survival rate was higher in the study group (Table 2) [31,34–40]. Subgroup analysis found survival rates of 52% and 25%, respectively, in treated and untreated patients who had gross serosal invasion, but subset analysis should be viewed cautiously. There was, however, a notable difference in peritoneal recurrence: 19 of the treated patients and 37 of the untreated patients had recurrent disease in the peritoneal cavity ($P = .03$). The study authors concluded that an intra-operative finding of gross serosal invasion may be used as a selection criterion for intraperitoneal chemotherapy.

Continuous hyperthermic peritoneal perfusion (CHPP) was designed to favorably alter the distribution and kinetics of agents used in IP chemotherapy [41]. A number of randomized trials of adjuvant CHPP have been performed in Japan and Korea (see Table 2). A pilot study by Yonemura and colleagues [41] investigated the role of this technique in 41 patients who had peritoneal dissemination. The 3-year survival rate was 28.5%; however, second-look laparotomy confirmed the reduction of carcinomatosis, and in half of the patients, ascites disappeared. In a follow-up study [42], the same group studied 139 patients who had T2 or

Table 2
Selected trials of intraperitoneal chemotherapy

Treatment groups	Stage	No. of patients	Survival rate (%)	P value	Reference
Cisplatin	T3–4 NXb	31	38 at 2 years	NS	[31]
Surgery alone		34	30 at 2 years		
Cisplatin	T 3–4 and M0	33	21 at 5 years	NS	[34]
Surgery alone		34	24 at 5 years		
Carbon-adsorbed MMC	T3–4 NX M0	24	69 at 3 years	<0.01	[35]
Surgery alone		25	27 at 3 years		
Carbon-adsorbed MMC	T3–4 NX	46	Closed early	NS	[36]
Surgery alone		45	Closed early		
MMC + 5-Fu	T1–4 N1–2 M0	125	54 at 5 years	0.02	[37]
Surgery alone		123	30 at 5 years		
CHPP (MMC)	T3 NX M0	42	64 at 5 years	NS	[38]
Surgery alone		40	52 at 5 years		
CHPP (MMC) + MMC + UFT	T3 NXb	77	51 at 5 years	NS	[39]
MMC + UFT		94	46 at 5 years		
CHPP (cisplatin + MMC)	T3 NX	22	68 at 3 years	<0.01	[40]
CHPP (cisplatin + MMC)		18	51 at 3 years		
Surgery alone		18	23 at 3 years		

Abbreviation: CHPP, continuous hyperthermic peritoneal perfusion.

greater disease. Patients were randomly assigned to receive either hyperthermic or normothermic intraperitoneal chemotherapy (mitomycin and cisplatin) versus surgery alone [3]. The overall 5-year survival rate was 61% in the hyperthermic group, 43% in the normothermic group, and 41% in the surgery only group. Heated IP chemotherapy was an independent predictor of improved survival after curative gastrectomy. As part of a Phase I study of IP hyperthermic perfusion at the authors' institution, 12 patients who had gastric cancer underwent this approach. Survival was significantly longer for patients who underwent IP hyperthermic perfusion than for a nonrandomized group of patients who had Stage IV disease and who were candidates for perfusion during the same period but elected to receive systemic chemotherapy. There were, unfortunately, two (17%) operative deaths in the treatment group, and all patients eventually succumbed to their disease.

Chemoradiotherapy

Moertel and colleagues [43] first investigated adjuvant 5-FU-based chemoradiation in the 1960s. A randomized trial was conducted comparing resection followed by observation with resection followed by postoperative chemoradiation (37.5 Gy with bolus 5-FU at 15 mg/kg for 3 days). By design, informed consent was obtained after randomization, and patients were not stratified for known prognostic factors. Ten of 39 patients refused adjuvant therapy after randomization. The local-regional control, overall survival, and relapse-free survival rates were all higher in the adjuvant therapy arm. Curiously, the overall survival rate was highest in the subgroup that refused chemoradiation after randomization. When analyzed by treatment actually received, survival was not statistically different. This study illustrates the problems that can arise in clinical trials with small numbers of patients, the importance of stratification for known prognostic variables, and the importance of obtaining consent for treatment before randomization.

Postoperative radiotherapy alone has also been investigated. The British Stomach Cancer Group conducted a Phase III trial that stratified 436 patients by age, symptom duration, and stage, and then randomized them to surgery alone, surgery followed by FAM chemotherapy (5-FU, doxorubicin, mitomycin), or surgery followed by radiotherapy (45 Gy in 25 fractions $\pm$ a 5.4 Gy boost) [22]. A local-regional control advantage was demonstrated in the radiotherapy arm, in spite of the fact that 18% of patients had positive margins and one third received 40 Gy or less (90%, versus 73% for surgery alone and 81% for surgery followed by chemotherapy; $P < 0.01$). The 5-year survival rate was 20% for surgery alone, 12% for surgery plus radiotherapy, and 19% for surgery plus chemotherapy. Cause-specific and overall survival rates were not statistically different. The investigators concluded that surgery should remain standard treatment for gastric cancer, and that adjuvant therapy should be used only under the auspices of a clinical trial. Even though a chemoradiation arm was not included, the failure of the study to show a difference in survival influenced their decision to subsequently investigate adjuvant chemotherapy alone in gastric cancer.

Several single-institution studies have also reported an advantage with postoperative radiotherapy, with or without concurrent chemotherapy [10,44–48]. One such trial from Spain [47] evaluated the role of adjuvant radiotherapy in patients who had high-risk gastric cancer. Sixty-two patients who had adverse clinical features, defined as serosal or regional nodal involvement, were randomized to receive surgical resection with intent to cure and external-beam radiotherapy, with or without intraoperative radiotherapy (IORT). Although the IORT group had a higher operative mortality rate, the relapse-free survival rate was similar in both groups, with a slight trend toward improved local control in the IORT group (11% versus 20%; $P < 0.3$). Although the number of patients is small, this study suggests that IORT might decrease the incidence of local recurrence.

The Gastrointestinal Intergroup recently reported the results of a large randomized trial (INT 0116) comparing postoperative chemoradiation with bolus 5-FU and 45 Gy radiation to complete surgical resection alone [10]. The study included patients who had a complete resection of a gastric or gastroesophageal junction tumor. The adjuvant regimen included chemotherapy administered before and after radiotherapy [49]. Radiation was administered to the tumor bed, regional nodes, and 2 cm beyond the proximal and distal margin of resection (45 Gy in 25 fractions). A total of 556 patients were evaluable (more than 600 entered the study). At a median follow-up of 5 years, the median survival duration of the chemoradiation group was 36 months versus 27 months for the surgery-alone group ($P = .005$). At 3 years, there was a 9% absolute (28% relative) survival advantage (50% versus 41%) in the postoperative chemoradiation arm, at the cost of significant gastrointestinal (33%) and hematologic (54%) toxic effects and a 1% incidence of treatment-related mortality. The treated group had a 19% local-regional failure rate, which was significantly less than that of the control group but still leaves room for improvement. It was reported that in approximately 30% of patients in the chemoradiation arm, a radiotherapy planning error occurred, and in 10% of patients, the error was potentially life-threatening. Such errors were corrected by a centralized quality assurance effort. For many, but not all, this trial establishes postoperative adjuvant fluorouracil-based chemoradiation as the standard of care in patients who have resected gastric cancer. Box 1 lists the regimen used in this study and to be considered for patients who have undergone complete resection.

There are, however, several concerns with this study [10]. Most important, the extent of surgical resection was not controlled, and the proportion of patients who did not recover quickly enough from surgical resection to undergo treatment is unknown (but has been estimated as 30% in other studies). In addition, pathologic evaluation failed to reveal any

---

Box 1. Gastrointestinal intergroup postoperative chemoradiotherapy regimen for patients with Stage Ib–IV disease after R0 resection

Chemotherapy (one 28-day cycle)
5-FU 425 mg/m^2/d intravenous (IV) on days 1–5
Folinic acid 20 mg/m^2/d IV on days 1–5

Chemoradiotherapy (5 weeks)
5-FU 400 mg/m^2/d IV on days 1–4 and on the last 3 days
   of radiotherapy
Folinic acid 20 mg/m^2/d IV on days 1–4 and on the last 3 days
   of radiotherapy
External-beam irradiation, 45 Gy at 1.8 Gy per day,
   5 days per week
1-month recovery period

Chemotherapy (two 28-day cycles)
5-FU 425 mg/m^2/d IV on days 1–5
Folinic acid 20 mg/m^2/d IV on days 1–5

lymph nodes in the resected specimens of over half the patients. Thus, many critics of this study suggest that the adjuvant treatment was simply making up for inadequate surgery.

Neoadjuvant therapy

Neoadjuvant therapy may be chemotherapy, radiotherapy, or a combination of modalities. Several potential advantages make preoperative therapy an attractive path for investigation and patient management. The biology of gastric tumors predisposes patients to micrometastatic disease at the time of presentation (based on a high treatment failure rate). Thus, neoadjuvant therapy may expose these cells to treatment when the cell growth fraction is high and the tumor volume is relatively low. Early initiation of systemic therapy may therefore eliminate these micrometastases. The ability to assess tumor response also may enable the early termination of ineffective therapy. In addition, preoperative therapy can downstage the primary gastric tumor and potentially improve the likelihood of a microscopically negative resection, and some patients who have occult chemoresistant metastasis that manifests during treatment and very aggressive disease may avoid nontherapeutic laparotomy. Preoperative therapy can also add prognostic information. An analysis of 83 patients who had gastric cancer treated on preoperative chemotherapy protocols at MD Anderson [50] showed that responders had a higher 5-year survival rate than nonresponders (83% versus 31%; $P < 0.001$). In fact, on multivariate analysis, response to preoperative chemotherapy was found to be the single most important predictor of survival. Preoperative approaches must be balanced by the potential risk of delaying definitive local therapy, however, particularly in early-stage tumors. Resistant clones theoretically may develop during therapy, and performance status may improve if initially poor nutritional status is reversed, or may deteriorate as a result of therapy and thus increase surgical risk.

Accurate clinical staging is essential in preoperative clinical trials. Because of the potential for downstaging, pretreatment endoscopic sonography and laparoscopy of all enrolled patients are encouraged for comparison with control groups. A number of chemotherapy regimens have been studied in small, Phase II preoperative trials, but heterogeneous patient selection and treatment plans make their results difficult to compare. They generally show that preoperative therapy is feasible and may downstage tumors, however. Well-designed Phase III trials are still needed.

Preoperative chemotherapy

Several clinical trials of preoperative chemotherapy in the management of gastric cancer have been attempted. Wilke and coworkers [51] first reported

34 patients who had unresectable disease at surgical exploration. The patients then underwent chemotherapy with a combination of etoposide, doxorubicin, and cisplatin, and subsequent re-exploration. The study authors found a pathologic complete response rate of 15%. This study demonstrated the feasibility of using neoadjuvant chemotherapy in advanced gastric cancer. Subsequent trials have been based on regimens using various combinations of etoposide, fluorouracil, cisplatin, doxorubicin and folinic acid, methotrexate, mitomycin, and interferon alpha [52–58]. The median survival duration in these studies ranges from 15 months to more than 4 years. The percentage of patients undergoing a microscopically negative resection ranges from 33% to 88%. Complete pathologic responses were noted and found to occur in 0% to 9% of patients. Trials that included more than 20 patients per treatment arm and evaluated the post-treatment outcome and median survival duration of patients undergoing subtotal or total gastrectomy after neoadjuvant chemotherapy are summarized in Table 3 [52–62].

At MD Anderson, the authors' group has studied neoadjuvant approaches for the management of this disease since the 1980s [50,53,58]. Our experience with neoadjuvant therapy progressed from an initial two cycles of preoperative therapy (etoposide, 5-FU, and leucovorin) to up to five preoperative cycles in patients who had responsive tumors. The last completed protocol of neoadjuvant chemotherapy alone consisted of 5-FU, cisplatin, and interferon [58]. Patients whose tumors demonstrated a response continued treatment for a total of five cycles of therapy. Upper gastrointestinal series, computed tomography, endoscopy, and pathologic evaluation were employed to assess response to treatment. Almost half of the patients received all five courses of preoperative chemotherapy, and 83% had an R0 resection. A pathologic complete response was noted in 7% of patients, and three additional patients had only microscopic carcinoma in the specimen. Median survival duration was 30 months. At Memorial Sloan Kettering Cancer Center, Kelsen and colleagues [56] combined neoadjuvant systemic chemotherapy with postoperative intraperitoneal therapy in 56 patients. The pathologic complete response rates were not recorded, but a grossly negative resection was achieved in more than 60% of the patients, and the median survival duration was 15 months.

A Phase II study by Ott and coworkers [63] evaluated the toxicity and efficacy of neoadjuvant cisplatin, fluorouracil, and leucovorin in locally advanced gastric cancer, with the hope of administering two cycles of therapy followed by surgery. Eighty-six percent of the 42 patients enrolled completed at least one cycle. Seventy-six percent of patients had resectable disease upon exploration, and after complete resection, the median survival duration was 32 months. Unfortunately, the incidence of peritoneal recurrence was relatively high at 62.5%.

The only completed and reported prospective randomized trial of neoadjuvant chemotherapy is a small study from the Dutch Gastric Cancer

Table 3
Selected trials of preoperative chemotherapy

Preoperative	Postoperative	Selection	No. of patients	R0	Median survival (months)	Pathologic CR	Ref
EFP × 2	EFP × 3	M0	25	72%	15	0	[52]
EAP × 3	EAP × 2	M0	48	77%	16	0	[53]
EAP × 3	EAP × 1	III–IV; M0	30	80%	17	0	[54]
EAP × 3	EAP × 3	II–III, M0	25	80%	>40	0	[59]
FU + cisplatin × 1–6	None	N + M0, >7 cm, Cardia tumor	30	59%	16	0	[55]
FU + FA + cisplatin × 2	IP FUDR + IP cisplatin × 1	Resectable	59	71%	>48	5 (9%)	[60]
EAFPLG	None	Unresectable, M0	82	45%	17	4 (5%)	[61]
FAMTX × 3	FU + IP cisplatin + IP 5-FU × 3	T3–4 NX M0 T2 N1–2 M0	56	61%	15	Not stated	[56]
FAMTX vs. none	None	T2–T4 M0	27 / 29	33% / 55%	18 / 30	0	[62]
PMUE	PMUE	IV	29	79%	NS[a]	0	[57]
None	PMUE		26	88%	NS		
5-FU + INF + cisplatin × 5	None	M0	30	83%	30	2 (7%)	[58]

[a] Overall median survival not stated; only subgroup analyses were reported.

Abbreviations: CR, complete response; EAFPLG, epi-doxorubicin, 5-FU, cisplatin, leucovorin, and glutathione; EAP, etoposide, doxorubicin, and cisplatin; EFP, etoposide, fluorouracil, and cisplatin; FA, folinic acid; FAMTX, fluorouracil, doxorubicin, and methotrexate; FU, fluorouracil; FUDR, 5-fluoro-2'-deoxyuridine; INF, interferon alfa-2b; PMUE, cisplatin, mitomycin, etoposide, and uracil-tegafur.

Group [64]. After the exclusion of patients who had metastatic disease, this study had only 20 patients in each arm, was clearly underpowered, and was a negative study. The German European Organization for Research and Treatment of Cancer (EORTC) trial [65] is an ongoing, well-designed, randomized trial. In this study, patients are being randomized to undergo surgery alone or preoperative cisplatin, 5-FU, and leucovorin followed by surgery. Initial Phase II work on this trial completed by Siewart and colleagues [65] evaluated the efficacy of a similar regimen. The Siewart group enrolled 41 patients, 36 of whom underwent surgical resection. Their complete resection rate was 73.2%, comparable to that of Ott and colleagues. After a median follow-up of almost 20 months, 73% of patients demonstrated no evidence of recurrent disease. On the basis of these data, the EORTC is now actively enrolling patients in a large, prospective, randomized clinical trial of neoadjuvant therapy using 5-FU, leucovorin, and cisplatin versus surgery alone.

The use of perioperative chemotherapy in patients who have resectable gastric and esophago-gastric cancer has been investigated recently in a large randomized clinical trial from the United Kingdom, termed the MRC (Medical Research Council) Adjuvant Gastric Infusional Chemotherapy (MAGIC) trial [66]. The investigators randomly assigned more than 500 patients to receive epirubicin, cisplatin, and infusional 5-FU during three preoperative and three postoperative cycles, or surgery alone. In the chemotherapy arm, 88% of patients completed preoperative chemotherapy, 55% commenced postoperative chemotherapy, and 40% completed all six cycles. The main reasons for failing to start postoperative chemotherapy were death, disease progression, patient request, and postoperative complications. A curative resection was achieved in 79% of chemotherapy patients compared with 69% who underwent surgery alone ($P = .02$). Postoperative morbidity and mortality rates were similar. The final survival analysis will be reported in the next several months.

Preoperative radiotherapy

Radiotherapy has been used successfully in the management of several types of malignancies. The earliest studies of radiotherapy for gastric cancer completed in the 1960s were not undertaken with curative intent. In 1998, Zhang and coworkers [67] reported the results of a large, prospective, randomized trial of neoadjuvant radiotherapy for patients who had resectable cancer of the gastric cardia. Three hundred and seventy patients were enrolled, and 171 received radiation at 40 Gy to the cardia, lower esophagus, fundus, and hepatogastric ligament. Gastric resection was undertaken 2 to 4 weeks later. Compared with the remaining 199 patients who underwent surgery alone, the radiotherapy plus surgery group had a significantly higher 5-year survival rate (30.1% versus 19.8%). Also, the operative mortality rate in the radiotherapy group was unexpectedly lower (0.6% versus 2.5%). Local-regional disease control was significantly better in the treatment group as well. The investigators concluded that preoperative radiotherapy improves survival in patients who have gastric cancer.

Preoperative chemoradiotherapy

Numerous studies have demonstrated a significant improvement in the effectiveness of radiotherapy when it is combined with chemotherapy for the treatment of tumors of the rectum as well as other sites. Combined-modality chemoradiotherapy in the preoperative setting allows for treatment with the target organ in place, which, compared with postoperative radiotherapy, may reduce radiotoxicity to the bowel and other adjacent organs. Preoperative radiotherapy with and without chemotherapy has been reported to improve outcomes in single-arm, single-institution experiences [68–71], and has been evaluated in prospective, randomized trials [72]. These trials demonstrated that suboptimal radiation doses without concurrent chemotherapy increased resectability and survival without increasing morbidity.

The Gastrointestinal Tumor Study Group used split-course radiotherapy (50 Gy) given with 5-FU, followed by maintenance 5-FU, methotrexate, and lomustine for patients who had locally advanced, unresectable gastric cancer [73]. This regimen resulted in a 4-year survival rate of 18%, compared with 6% for radiotherapy alone. In the 1990s, the authors began a pilot study of neoadjuvant chemoradiotherapy (combined with IORT) for patients who have gastric cancer that was determined to be potentially resectable using a combination of computed tomography, endoscopic ultrasonography, and staging laparoscopy [74]. The treatment combined 45 Gy of external-beam radiation at 1.8 Gy per day, 5 days per week with continuous-infusion 5-FU ($300 \text{ mg/m}^2/\text{d}$). Twenty-four patients who had potentially resectable but poor-prognosis tumors (determined by endoscopic ultrasonography [EUS] to be T2 or higher) were treated, and all but one patient were able to complete the therapy. The radiation field included the entire stomach and regional lymph nodes. Patients were restaged on the basis of a computed tomography scan at 4 to 6 weeks following treatment and before a planned resection. A spleen-preserving D-2 gastrectomy was performed after completion of chemoradiotherapy in 19 (83%) patients. Intraoperative radiotherapy (10 Gy) was given at resection. Complete pathologic response was observed in 2 (11%) patients. Soon after the feasibility of this study was established, a larger Phase II trial was begun. The preliminary results of the two studies were reported in abstract form. Of the 44 patients enrolled at that time, 39 had successfully completed EUS, and all were stage T2 or higher (82% were T3 or T4). Forty-three patients completed chemoradiation. Upon restaging, 9 patients (20%) were found to have distant disease and did not require a palliative surgical procedure. Thirty-two (73%)

patients underwent resection; 2 patients refused resection. Five (11%) patients had a pathologic complete response, whereas 18 (41%) patients had partial responses with evidence of downstaging compared with preoperative EUS results. There was one postoperative death, and 4 patients required reoperation. There were four symptomatic leaks, two esophageal and two duodenal stump leaks. With a minimum follow-up of 9 months, the overall median survival duration was 34 months, with the disease-specific survival rate being higher than 60% at 4 years in resected patients. These encouraging results led to the approach of induction chemotherapy incorporating newer agents, followed by fluorouracil-based chemoradiotherapy in the preoperative setting.

In a recent study at MD Anderson [75], the authors' group treated patients with two courses of 5-FU, folinic acid, and cisplatin and followed that with 5-FU-potentiated radiotherapy (45 Gy). Surgical resection after preoperative chemoradiotherapy was performed without excessive complications. Thirty-four patients who had localized gastric adenocarcinoma were enrolled in the study, and 85% underwent resection. The pathologic complete response rate was 30%, and a partial response was seen in 24% of patients. The overall median survival duration was 33.7 months; however, patients who achieved a complete response had a median survival duration of 64 months, versus 12.6 months in those who had less than a complete response ($P < 0.05$). This study emphasizes that a durable survival benefit can be achieved in patients whose tumors respond to treatment.

Summary

The incidence of gastric cancer in the United States is decreasing; however, this disease still results in considerable mortality. Although effective surgical resection abiding by accepted oncologic principles allows for the highest probability of a cure, additional therapy in the form of neoadjuvant or adjuvant techniques may improve survival and quality of life. Well-designed prospective randomized trials are needed to determine whether the addition of new antineoplastic agents, the use of inhibitors of angiogenesis, or preoperative as opposed to postoperative therapy will further improve survival rates for this disease.

References

[1] Haenszel W. Variation in incidence of and mortality from stomach cancer, with particular reference to the United States. J Natl Cancer Inst 1958;21:213–62.
[2] Surveillance, Epidemiology, and End Results (SEER) program, public use data (1975–2001). Available at: http://seer.cancer.gov/faststats/. Accessed June 28, 2005.
[3] Wiggins CL, Becker TM, Key CR, et al. Stomach cancer among New Mexico's American Indians, Hispanic whites, and non-Hispanic whites. Cancer Res 1989;49:1595–9.
[4] Pisani P, Parkin DM, Bray F, et al. Estimates of the worldwide mortality from 25 cancers in 1990. Int J Cancer 1999;83:18–29.

[5] Parkin DM, Pisani P, Ferlay J. Global cancer statistics. CA Cancer J Clin 1999;49:33–64.

[6] Esaki Y, Hirayama R, Hirokawa K. A comparison of patterns of metastasis in gastric cancer by histologic type and age. Cancer 1990;65:2086–90.

[7] Maehara Y, Moriguchi S, Kakeji Y, et al. Pertinent risk factors and gastric carcinoma with synchronous peritoneal dissemination or liver metastasis. Surgery 1991; 110:820–3.

[8] Yao JC, Schnirer II, Reddy S, et al. Effects of sex and racial/ethnic group on the pattern of gastric cancer localization. Gastric Cancer 2002;5:208–12.

[9] Hundahl SA, Phillips JL, Menck HR. The National Cancer Data Base report on poor survival of US gastric carcinoma patients treated with gastrectomy: 5th edition. American Joint Committee on Cancer staging, proximal disease, and the "different disease" hypothesis. Cancer 2000;88:921–32.

[10] Macdonald JS, Smalley S, Benedetti J, et al. Chemotherapy after surgery compared with surgery alone for adenocarcinoma of the stomach or gastroesophageal junction. N Engl J Med 2001;345:725–30.

[11] Yao JC, Shimada K, Ajani JA. Adjuvant therapy for gastric carcinoma: closing out the century. Oncology (Huntingt) 1999;13:1485–94 [discussion: 1497–502].

[12] Earle CC, Maroun JA. Adjuvant chemotherapy after curative resection for gastric cancer in non-Asian patients: revisiting a meta-analysis of randomised trials. Eur J Cancer 1999;35: 1059–64.

[13] Janunger KG, Hafstrom L, Nygren P, et al. A systematic overview of chemotherapy effects in gastric cancer. Acta Oncol 2001;40:309–26.

[14] Imanaga H, Nakazato H. Results of surgery for gastric cancer and effect of adjuvant mitomycin C on cancer recurrence. World J Surg 1977;2:213–21.

[15] Grau JJ, Estape J, Alcobendas F, et al. Positive results of adjuvant mitomycin-C in resected gastric cancer: a randomised trial on 134 patients. Eur J Cancer 1993;29A:340–2.

[16] Gastrointestinal Tumor Study Group. A comparison of combination chemotherapy and combined modality therapy for locally advanced gastric carcinoma. Cancer 1982;49: 1116–22.

[17] Higgins GA, Amadeo JH, Smith DE, et al. Efficacy of prolonged intermittent therapy with combined 5-FU and methyl-CCNU following resection for gastric carcinoma. A Veterans Administration Surgical Oncology Group report. Cancer 1983;52:1105–12.

[18] Engstrom PF, Lavin PT, Douglass HO Jr, et al. Postoperative adjuvant 5-fluorouracil plus mehyl-CCNU therapy for gastric cancer patients. Eastern Cooperative Oncology Group study (EST 3275). Cancer 1985;55:1868–73.

[19] Macdonald JS, Fleming TR, Peterson RF, et al. Adjuvant chemotherapy with 5-FU, adriamycin, and mitomycin-C (FAM) versus surgery alone for patients with locally advanced gastric adenocarcinoma: a Southwest Oncology Group study. Ann Surg Oncol 1995;2:488–94.

[20] Lise M, Nitti D, Marchet A, et al. Final results of a Phase III clinical trial of adjuvant chemotherapy with the modified fluorouracil, doxorubicin, and mitomycin regimen in resectable gastric cancer. J Clin Oncol 1995;13:2757–63.

[21] Coombes RC, Schein PS, Chilvers CE, et al. A randomized trial comparing adjuvant fluorouracil, doxorubicin, and mitomycin with no treatment in operable gastric cancer. International Collaborative Cancer Group. J Clin Oncol 1990;8:1362–9.

[22] Hallissey MT, Dunn JA, Ward LC, et al. The second British Stomach Cancer Group trial of adjuvant radiotherapy or chemotherapy in resectable gastric cancer: five-year follow-up. Lancet 1994;343:1309–12.

[23] Krook JE, O'Connell MJ, Wieand HS, et al. A prospective, randomized evaluation of intensive-course 5-fluorouracil plus doxorubicin as surgical adjuvant chemotherapy for resected gastric cancer. Cancer 1991;67:2454–8.

[24] Neri B, de Leonardis V, Romano S, et al. Adjuvant chemotherapy after gastric resection in node-positive cancer patients: a multicentre randomised study. Br J Cancer 1996;73:549–52.

[25] Allum WH, Hallissey MT, Kelly KA. Adjuvant chemotherapy in operable gastric cancer. 5 year follow-up of first British Stomach Cancer Group trial. Lancet 1989;1:571–4.

[26] Grau JJ, Estape J, Fuster J, et al. Randomized trial of adjuvant chemotherapy with mitomycin plus ftorafur versus mitomycin alone in resected locally advanced gastric cancer. J Clin Oncol 1998;16:1036–9.

[27] Carrato A, Diaz-Rubio E, Medrano J, et al. Phase III trial of surgery versus adjuvant chemotherapy with mitomycin C (MMC) and tegafur plus uracil (UFT), starting within the first week after surgery, for gastric adenocarcinoma [abstract]. In: Proceedings of the Annual Meeting of the American Society for Clininical Oncolology; 1995. p. A468.

[28] The Italian Gastrointestinal Tumor Study Group. Adjuvant treatments following curative resection for gastric cancer. Br J Surg 1988;75:1100–4.

[29] Jakesz R, Dittrich C, Funovics J, et al. The effect of adjuvant chemotherapy in gastric carcinoma is dependent on tumor histology: 5-year results of a prospective randomized trial. Recent Results Cancer Res 1988;110:44–51.

[30] Kim JP, Kwon OJ, Oh ST, et al. Results of surgery on 6589 gastric cancer patients and immunochemosurgery as the best treatment of advanced gastric cancer. Ann Surg 1992;216: 269–78 [discussion: 278–9].

[31] Nakajima T, Nashimoto A, Kitamura M, et al. Adjuvant mitomycin and fluorouracil followed by oral uracil plus tegafur in serosa-negative gastric cancer: a randomized trial. Lancet 1999;354:273–7.

[32] Higgins GA Jr, Amadeo JH, McElhinney J, et al. Efficacy of prolonged intermittent therapy with combined 5-fluorouracil and methyl-CCNU following resection for carcinoma of the large bowel. A Veterans Administration Surgical Oncology Group report. Cancer 1984;53: 1–8.

[33] Schiessel R, Funovics J, Schick B, et al. Adjuvant intraperitoneal cisplatin therapy in patients with operated gastric carcinoma: results of a randomized trial. Acta Med Austriaca 1989;6: 68–9.

[34] Sautner T, Hofbauer F, Depisch D, et al. Adjuvant intraperitoneal cisplatin chemotherapy does not improve long-term survival after surgery for advanced gastric cancer. J Clin Oncol 1994;12:970–4.

[35] Hagiwara A, Takahashi T, Kojima O, et al. Prophylaxis with carbon-adsorbed mitomycin against peritoneal recurrence of gastric cancer. Lancet 1992;339:629–31.

[36] Rosen HR, Jatzko G, Repse S, et al. Adjuvant intraperitoneal chemotherapy with carbon-adsorbed mitomycin in patients with gastric cancer: results of a randomized multicenter trial of the Austrian Working Group for Surgical Oncology. J Clin Oncol 1998;16:2733–8.

[37] Yu W, Whang I, Chung H, et al. Indications for early postoperative intraperitioneal chemotherapy of advanced gastric cancer: results of a prospective randomized trial. World J Surg 2001;25:985–90.

[38] Hamazoe R, Maeta M, Kaibara N. Intraperitoneal thermochemotherapy for prevention of peritoneal recurrence of gastric cancer. Final results of a randomized controlled study. Cancer 1994;73:2048–52.

[39] Ikeguchi M, Kondou A, Oka A, et al. Effects of continuous hyperthermic peritoneal perfusion on prognosis of gastric cancer with serosal invasion. Eur J Surg 1995;161:581–6.

[40] Fujimura T, Yonemura Y, Muraoka K, et al. Continuous hyperthermic peritoneal perfusion for the prevention of peritoneal recurrence of gastric cancer: randomized controlled study. World J Surg 1994;18:150–5.

[41] Yonemura Y, Fujimura T, Fushida S, et al. Hyperthermo-chemotherapy combined with cytoreductive surgery for the treatment of gastric cancer with peritoneal dissemination. World J Surg 1991;15:530–5 [discussion: 535–6].

[42] Yonemura Y, de Aretxabala X, Fujimura T, et al. Intraoperative chemohyperthermic peritoneal perfusion as an adjuvant to gastric cancer: final results of a randomized controlled trial. Hepatogastroenterology 2001;48:1776–82.

[43] Moertel CG, Childs DS Jr, Reitemeier RJ, et al. Combined 5-fluorouracil and supervoltage radiation therapy of locally unresectable gastrointestinal cancer. Lancet 1969;2:865–7.

[44] Robinson E, Cohen Y. The combination of surgery, radiotherapy, and chemotherapy in the treatment of gastric cancer. Recent Results Cancer Res 1977;177–80.

[45] Regine WF, Mohiuddin M. Impact of adjuvant therapy on locally advanced adenocarcinoma of the stomach. Int J Radiat Oncol Biol Phys 1992;24:921–7.

[46] Slot A, Meerwaldt JH, van Putten WL, et al. Adjuvant postoperative radiotherapy for gastric carcinoma with poor prognostic signs. Radiother Oncol 1989;16:269–74.

[47] Martinez-Monge R, Calvo FA, Azinovic I, et al. Patterns of failure and long-term results in high-risk resected gastric cancer treated with postoperative radiotherapy with or without intraoperative electron boost. J Surg Oncol 1997;66:24–9.

[48] Gez E, Sulkes A, Yablonsky-Peretz T, et al. Combined 5-fluorouracil (5-FU) and radiation therapy following resection of locally advanced gastric carcinoma. J Surg Oncol 1986;31: 139–42.

[49] Poon MA, O'Connell MJ, Moertel CG, et al. Biochemical modulation of fluorouracil: evidence of significant improvement of survival and quality of life of patients with advanced colorectal carcinoma. J Clin Oncol 1989;7:1407–18.

[50] Lowy AM, Mansfield PF, Leach SD, et al. Response to neoadjuvant chemotherapy best predicts survival after curative resection of gastric cancer. Ann Surg 1999;229:303–8.

[51] Wilke H, Presser P, Fink U, et al. Preoperative chemotherapy in locally advanced and nonresectable gastric cancer: a Phase II study of etoposide, doxorubicin and cisplatin. J Clin Oncol 1989;7:1318–26.

[52] Ajani JA, Ota DM, Jessup JM, et al. Resectable gastric carcinoma. An evaluation of preoperative and postoperative chemotherapy. Cancer 1991;68:1501–6.

[53] Ajani JA, Mayer RJ, Ota DM, et al. Preoperative and postoperative combination chemotherapy for potentially resectable gastric carcinoma. J Natl Cancer Inst 1993;85: 1839–44.

[54] Fink U, Schuhmacher C, Stein HJ, et al. Preoperative chemotherapy for Stage III–IV gastric carcinoma: feasibility, response and outcome after complete resection. Br J Surg 1995;82: 1248–52.

[55] Rougier P, Mahjoubi M, Lasser P, et al. Neoadjuvant chemotherapy in locally advanced gastric carcinoma—a Phase II trial with combined continuous intravenous 5-fluorouracil and bolus cisplatinum. Eur J Cancer 1994;30A:1269–75.

[56] Kelsen D, Karpeh M, Schwartz G, et al. Neoadjuvant therapy of high-risk gastric cancer: a Phase II trial of preoperative FAMTX and postoperative intraperitoneal fluorouracil-cisplatin plus intravenous fluorouracil. J Clin Oncol 1996;14:1818–28.

[57] Yonemura Y, Sawa T, Kinoshita K, et al. Neoadjuvant chemotherapy for high-grade advanced gastric cancer. World J Surg 1993;17:256–61.

[58] Ajani JA, Mansfield PF, Lynch PM, et al. Enhanced staging and all chemotherapy preoperatively in patients with potentially resectable gastric carcinoma. J Clin Oncol 1999; 17:2403–11.

[59] Barone C, Cassano A, Pozzo C, et al. Long term follow up of a pilot Phase II study with neoadjuvant epidoxorubicin, etoposide and cisplatin in gastric cancer. Oncology 2004;67: 48–53.

[60] Crookes P, Leichman CG, Leichman L, et al. Systemic chemotherapy for gastric carcinoma followed by postoperative intraperitoneal therapy: a final report. Cancer 1997;79:1767–75.

[61] Cascinu S, Scartozzi M, Labianca R, et al. High curative resection rate with weekly cisplatin, 5-fluorouracil, epidoxorubicin, 6S-leucovorin, glutathione, and filgastrim in patients with locally advanced, unresectable gastric cancer: a report from the Italian Group for the Study of Digestive Tract Cancer (GISCAD). Br J Cancer 2004;90:1521–5.

[62] Hartgrink HH, van de Velde CJ, Putter H, et al. Neo-adjuvant chemotherapy for operable gastric cancer: long term results of the Dutch randomised FAMTX trial. Eur J Surg Oncol 2004;30:643–9.

[63] Ott K, Sendler A, Becker K, et al. Neoadjuvant chemotherapy with cisplatin, 5-FU, and leucovorin in locally advanced gastric cancer: a prospective Phase II study. Gastric Cancer 2003;6:159–67.

[64] Songun I, Kaizer HJ, Hermans J, et al. Chemotherapy for operable gastric cancer: results of the Dutch randomized FAMTX trial. The Dutch Gastric Cancer Study Group. Eur J Cancer 1999;35:558–62.

[65] Siewart JR, Schumacher C, Fink U. The German EORTC study of neoadjuvant therapy of stomach carcinoma. Langenbecks Arch Chir Suppl Kongressbd 1998;115:717–9.

[66] Allum W, Cunningham D, Weeden S, et al. Perioperative chemotherapy in operable gastric and lower oesophageal cancer: a randomised, controlled trial (the MAGIC trial, ISRCTN 93793971) [abstract]. Proc Am Soc Clin Oncol 2003;22:249.

[67] Zhang ZX, Gu XZ, Yin WB, et al. Randomized clinical trial of the combination of preoperative irradiation and surgery in the treatment of adenocarcinoma of the gastric cardia (AGC)—report on 370 patients. Int J Radiat Oncol Biol Phys 1998;42:929–34.

[68] Groves LK, Rodriguez-Antunez A. Treatment of carcinoma of the esophagus and gastric cardia with concentrated preoperative irradiation followed by early operation. A progress report. Ann Thorac Surg 1973;5:333–8.

[69] Kamimura S, Mikuriya S, Hara O, et al. [Preoperative radiotherapy of carcinoma of the stomach and breast]. Gan to Kagaku Ryoho 1987;14:1558–63 [in Japanese].

[70] Mikuriya S, Oh'ami H. Radiotherapy and cellular infiltration of tumor nests. Radiat Med 1983;1:248–54.

[71] Yu W, Whang I, Averbach A, et al. Morbidity and mortality of early postoperative intraperitoneal chemotherapy as adjuvant therapy for gastric cancer. Am Surg 1998;64:1104–8.

[72] Shchepotin IB, Evans SR, Chorny V, et al. Intensive preoperative radiotherapy with local hyperthermia for the treatment of gastric carcinoma. Surg Oncol 1994;3:37–44.

[73] A comparison of combination chemotherapy and combination therapy for locally advanced gastric carcinoma. Gastrointestinal Tumor Study Group. Cancer 1982;49:1771–7.

[74] Lowy AM, Feig BW, Janjan N, et al. A pilot study of preoperative chemoradiotherapy for resectable gastric cancer. Ann Surg Oncol 2001;8:519–24.

[75] Ajani JA, Mansfield PF, Janjan N, et al. Multi-institutional trial of preoperative chemoradiotherapy in patients with potentially resectable gastric cancer. J Clin Oncol 2004;22:2774–80.

ELSEVIER
SAUNDERS

Surg Clin N Am 85 (2005) 1053–1059

SURGICAL
CLINICS OF
NORTH AMERICA

Index

Note: Page numbers of article titles are in **boldface** type.

0039-6109/05/$ - see front matter © 2005 Elsevier Inc. All rights reserved.
doi:10.1016/S0039-6109(05)00111-8   *surgical.theclinics.com*

S

Satiety, physiology of, 889

Selective vagotomy, for ulcer disease, 914, 925

Self-expanding endoluminal stents, for gastric cancer, 1012

Sentinel lymph node biopsy, for gastric cancer, 1023

Short esophagus, and antireflux surgery, 939–940

Stomach
    acid-peptic disorders of. *See* Acid-peptic disorders.
    anatomy of, 875–883, 967–968
        anatomic relationships in, 878–880
        arterial blood supply in, 880–881
        historical aspects of, 875–876
        innervation in, 882
        landmarks in, 876–878
            gastroesophageal junction, 876
        lymphatic drainage in, 882–883
    cancer of. *See* Gastric cancer.
    functional anatomy and physiology of, 884–892, 968–970
        accommodation, 968–969
        alkaline secretion by gastric mucosa, 886–887
        antropyloric coordination, 970
        emptying, 969–970
        evolving areas of interest in, 891–892
        gastric digestion and contribution to downstream absorption, 887–888
        gastric motility. *See* Gastric motility.
        gastric mucosa, 884
        gastroparesis. *See* Gastroparesis.
        in response to meal, 889–891
        neuroendocrine regulation of acid secretion, 884–886
        satiety, 889
        trituration, 969
    functional evaluation of, 970–972
        antroduodenal manometry in, 971
        electrogastrography in, 971
        solid phase gastric emptying scan in, 970–971
        upper endoscopy in, 970
        upper gastrointestinal series in, 970

Stretta procedure, for gastroesophageal reflux disease. *See* Endoscopic therapy.

Stromal tumors, gastrointestinal. *See* Gastrointestinal stromal tumors.

Sucralfate, for acid-peptic disorders, 901

T

Tegaserod, for gastroparesis, 981–982

TNM system, of staging, for gastric cancer, 1024

Total fundoplication, for gastroesophageal reflux disease, 935

Total parenteral nutrition, for gastroparesis, 983

Transgastric drainage, of pancreatic pseudocysts, 1000–1005

Transgastric resection
    of early gastric cancer, 993–996
    of gastrointestinal stromal tumors, 996, 998–1000

Transpyloric gastroduodenotomy, for bleeding duodenal ulcers, 910

Trituration, gastric, physiology of, 969

Truncal vagotomy, for ulcer disease, 914, 924–925

U

Ulcer disease. *See also* Acid-peptic disorders.
    classification of, 908
    hemorrhage in, 909–911
        Helicobacter pylori and, 911
        surgical management of, 915–916
            transpyloric gastroduodenotomy in, 910
    perforation of, 909
        Helicobacter pylori and, 909
    surgical management of, **907–929**
        Billroth procedures in, 917, 919, 921
            and bile gastritis, 921
        Braun enteroenterostomy in, 921
        for bleeding duodenal ulcers, 909–911
        for proximal gastric ulcers, 922–924
        highly selective vagotomy in, 914, 925
        omental patch in, 915
        partial gastrectomy and restoration of foregut continuity in, 917, 919, 921–924

Changing Your Address?

Make sure your subscription changes too! When you notify us of your new address, you can help make our job easier by including an exact copy of your Clinics label number with your old address (see illustration below.) This number identifies you to our computer system and will speed the processing of your address change. Please be sure this label number accompanies your old address and your corrected address—you can send an old Clinics label with your number on it or just copy it exactly and send it to the address listed below.

We appreciate your help in our attempt to give you continuous coverage. Thank you.

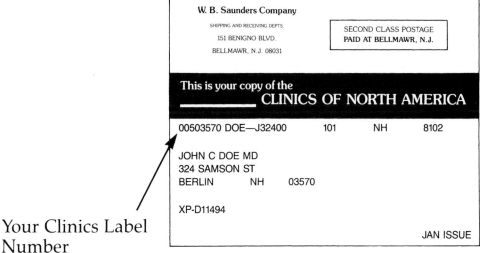

Your Clinics Label Number
Copy it exactly or send your label
along with your address to:
W.B. Saunders Company, Customer Service
Orlando, FL 32887-4800
Call Toll Free 1-800-654-2452

Please allow four to six weeks for delivery of new subscriptions and for processing address changes.